Swimming with Fishes

Rasheda Ashanti Malcolm

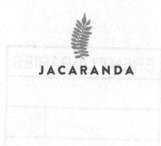

JACARANDA

First published in Great Britain 2017 by
Jacaranda Books Art Music Ltd
Unit 304 Metal Box Factory
30 Great Guildford Street,
London SE1 0HS
www.jacarandabooksartmusic.co.uk

A CIP catalogue record for this book is available from the
British Library

ISBN: 978-1-909762-45-9
eISBN: 978-1-909762-46-6

Printed and bound in Great Britain
by CPI Group (UK) Ltd, Croydon, CR0 4YY

For my beloved Mummy and Daddy

One

Katherine 'Kat' Lewis

Jamaica

Kat Lewis wanted a baby more than she wanted to live. Ever since her mother, Miss Ruthie, explained that she should never have a baby because of the risk it posed to her life. It didn't matter that folks told her any child she conceived would probably never survive, the slightest chance of success meant there was hope.

Kat had never been an observer of limits, and the restrictions put on her because of her illness were never adhered to, especially in her head. Her daily trek to the beach in protest against being constantly viewed as an invalid was especially true on this day, her twenty-eighth birthday.

Kat walked deep in thoughts, savouring the feel of the warm white sand between her toes, her sketch pad and pencils in a cloth bag flung over one shoulder while her flip-flops hung loosely between two fingers. Her hair, long, thick and black, was tied up in a ponytail away from her slim oval face, gently swinging from side to side as she walked. Her nose was straight and flared at the nostrils and when she smiled, her wide, full lips revealed a gap between her two top teeth. She had been told that she had inherited her father's brown eyes, huge and almond shaped, his proud angular chin and her mother's bronze, smooth skin. She was slender, no matter how much she ate, weight never stuck to her, one of a series of reasons why her health was such a concern to some Meadow folks, but she had curves in the right places and her walk was innate royalty.

With each step the soft-grains gave way beneath her bare feet. She shaded her eyes from the glare of the afternoon sun, which had transformed the beach into a sheet of shimmering silver. Some days it took a great deal for her to make these walks, but she did so religiously, making her way from her mother's house to the line where the road ended and the beach began. Only a crisis—a sickle cell attack—could prevent her daily trek, forcing her to take to her bed.

Kat was born with sickle cell anaemia. Her early childhood was a hazy mist of white hospital walls, doctors, morphine, drips, folic acid, penicillin and pain, rendering her a mere spectator of life. Like many people who've faced death and lived to tell the tale, she was fully appreciative of each second. This is the reason why her daily walks to the beach were so important. They gave her the chance to feel fully alive and often free from pain. She could watch children play and young pregnant women reclining on the beach, their bellies revealed, smooth and hard. She loved to watch those women the most, to marvel at the miracle happening inside of them, to hope, wish, dream and pray that one day she would have her own.

She had been like a sponge in water soaking up the

old adages of the folks in her small rural town regarding childless women. Over the years she had witnessed that no childless woman escaped ridicule or the malicious lash of the gossips' tongue as to the reasons God had withheld the fruit of her womb. The older women believed children were paramount to a holy marriage, that children somehow made it impossible for Satan to tempt a man away from his wife. The men also lived by this, even in the twenty-first century, and if their wife could not give them an offspring, then they were justified in maintaining a mistress who could provide a home for their seeds. This fable had gained cultural status among the folks in the Meadows, where everyone knew everyone and in the church yard your genealogy went back generations; and where things were always in-keeping with traditions.

The Meadows could easily be called Jamaica's forgotten gem, with its culture of retaining these old-fashioned ideologies. It was a small fishing village on the coastal west of the island, framed by the ocean and four miles of powdery white sand and scattered with trees of every kind; palm, coconut, almond, avocado. Turning off the main road led you onto the dusty lanes and into the hills, where goats and cows could be seen roaming along the roadside, independently or being led by their owner, who was usually a farmer. The town's main income came from fishing and tourism. God and the church was the glue of society and a respect that held the elders in high esteem was unwritten policy.

Kat had lived her whole life in the Meadows. She had gone to the best schools, where the majority of the teachers were white and the pupils came from wealthy families. Thanks to a trust fund left by her father for her education, Kat was able to study Art and Design at university. After graduating, she started selling her paintings, taking on commissions and teaching art at the local community centre to make a living.

Kat continued making her way to the far end of the beach where few tourists ventured. At her destination she sat cross-legged on a large flat piece of stone embedded in the sand, shaded by the huge leaves of two palm trees. The stone was smooth and warm from the sun's glow, as she knew it would be and she swore by its healing properties, feeling the heat spreading through her like a pan on a hot stove. Reaching for her bag she pulled out the sketch pad and pencils, her eyes scanning the area for possibilities. Afternoons were the busiest time of day on the beach. She observed the swarm of tourists from the hotels and guest houses, the vendors and natives coming up from the valley or down from the hills to sell their merchandise and memorabilia. The smell of the jerk chicken, and freshly seasoned fried fish was carried on the breeze to remind her to eat. The occasional group of tourists passed her. A smiling couple, a child with his father, both smeared with white cream to fend off the burning sun, and a very large white lady who had turned pink and was accompanied by the thinnest young boy whose meagre arms struggled to fit around her. Kat knew him. He was the Post Office mistress Nellie Potato's grandson and though it wouldn't show in him, he would surely eat well this day. Some of the young men of the Meadows discovered a way of making a living out of pleasuring middle-aged overweight, white and sometimes black tourists who were only too willing to pay for their services. The vulnerability of these seemingly affluent and professional women only went to confirm to Kat that women gave away everything for love.

Out of the blue her attention was caught by the gliding of a white and grey pelican as it swooped into the sea, emerging with its snack between its beak; a struggling fish that was swiftly swallowed.

'Pssssssssssst.'

Kat startled, hearing the hiss but unable to see anyone.

'It's me, Miss Kat.'

Old Man Jaguar, the beach attendant, emerged from behind a coconut tree. He was dressed as though he had been or was going to a very important event, with a creaseless khaki shirt matching his classic trousers. His salt and pepper hair shone with hair oil and was neatly parted to the right. His bushy silver eyebrows met in the middle, partly concealing small dark eyes. He gave Kat a wide, friendly grin, revealing a gold tooth at the top. She smiled. Old Man was always a welcome sight for her.

'Wishing you many happy returns, Miss Kat. Beg you a little of your time please. A word in your ears about Miss Rootie,' he whispered as if it were a secret.

'Oh, Old Man, come by the house later, you can talk to Miss Ruthie yourself.'

He flapped his arms in frustration. 'I pass by earlier, but she chase me away like a dawg with rabies.'

She stifled a laugh knowing what a tyrant her mother could be, but also fully aware of Old Man's adoration for Miss Ruthie. Her mother sold provisions from their front yard and Kat could not remember a time when Old Man did not pass by their home on the pretext of buying a few limes, onions or eggs. He came with the crack of dawn, her mother would complain, although Kat knew Miss Ruthie deep, deep down in her soul loved his company as much as she enjoyed playing out annoyance at his presence.

'You know how she is. Try again later, she may be in a better mood.'

Old Man didn't seem to know which way to turn and it became obvious to Kat that he had more to say.

'Twenty-eight… that's plenty time left for a husband and babies. God has his plans, don't you mind bad talk.'

Kat smiled knowingly. No doubt Old Man had been witness to some recent gossip surrounding 'poor' her, which was no surprise. She could imagine it: 'Poor Kat, with no chick nor child. Poor Miss Ruthie, no grans to look forward to.' Kat had become immune to this kind of talk. Most of the girls she went to school with had migrated to other countries, were married or living with partners and nearly all had families. Babies. No-one expected the same for her.

'You know bad talk doesn't affect me, Old Man, but thanks for the concern. See you later.'

Old Man walked away, one hand tucked deep in his pocket with the other swinging like a member of a military regiment. Suddenly Kat spotted a familiar generous figure in the distance, floating along with the grace of a catwalk model. She recognised Mother Cynthy, feared and revered by many because they believed her to be an *obeah* woman—a witch. As a child Kat was a frequent visitor to Mother Cynthy's house, tucked away in the hills to the east. Miss Ruthie had been taking her to see the lady who lived in a house painted half purple ever since she could remember. The joke told by town folks was that after Mother Cynthy's divorce, the judge had said her husband was entitled to half the house. So she divided the house in two, keeping the half with the kitchen and the bathroom and covered every wall and surface including the floor in her half, various shades of purple. In that slightly eerie house that always smelled of the forest, Kat was given hot herbal and bush baths to soothe her joints and both sweet and bitter tasting concoctions to drink with the promise that it would improve her health. And whatever Mother Cynthy put into those concoctions of hers, whenever Kat sensed a sickle attack coming and started sipping those weird tasting liquids, she was somehow elevated from her body until the diminishing pain allowed her back in.

She watched Mother Cynthy walk towards her with a huge basket balanced on her head filled with bush teas, mangos, avocado pears and herbal medicines wrapped in brown paper bags. Tied around her wide waist was an apron sprouting many pockets filled with more packages. Kat's eyes followed her movements as she removed the basket with ease and set it on the log. She then perched beside it and smiled with the knowledge of someone in possession of a great secret.

'Happy birt'day. I glad I live to see you reach twenty-eight! Plenty years is that, for a baby those fool-fool folks say would not live to see five.'

'Thank you.' Kat smiled, eager to hear Mother Cynthy's next words.

'The heat real today.' She wiped her brow with her hand and removed her red head tie to smooth back her shock of dyed red hair. Her earth dark skin gleamed and three beads of sweat settled on her broad nose.

'Summer comes earlier each year, Mother Cynthy—it can only get hotter. What secret are you holding? I can see that sly smile of yours.'

'How's Miss Rootie?' asked Mother Cynthy, deliberately ignoring Kat's insinuation. 'Still praying to sweet Jesus for a husband to keep you still, I bet.'

'You know my mother.'

'And still putting de fear of God in you to prevent you from ever having a child, I'm sure.'

Kat laughed, nodding, and repeated, 'You know my mother.'

'I also know I would find you here. You love this stone, eh. Been sitting on it and drawing pictures from you old enough to walk.' Mother Cynthy smiled with genuine affection. Years ago, when the whole town had thought Miss Ruthie would never have a child she had predicted Kat's conception.

'Yes, ma'am. Columbus says stones are like bones, indestructible. This one has powers.'

'It has whatever you believe it to have.' She liked the fact that Kat practiced intuition, so unlike the youngsters of today.

Kat loved conversing with the bush woman. Mother Cynthy wasn't one to ridicule a person's beliefs, since her own were so peculiar. Miss Ruthie said Mother Cynthy had Maroon blood, which you could tell from her smooth black skin. Her piercing wise eyes and her knowledge of herbal plants was extensive, passed down to her by her Maroon mother, who received it from her own mother before that.

'How you been, Kat? All is well in your world? Not

seen you for a while.'

'I've been right here, every afternoon, it's you who's been scarce.'

'Yes, that's true. I can't always take de tourists. They come and expect to take pictures of us like monkey in a zoo. I get too mad sometimes.'

'They don't mean no harm, they're just curious.'

'They don't mean no damn good either, they out to exploit!'

'Old Man says life's never been so good. He says plenty people have jobs now, more than when he was a boy. He says the twentieth, and now the twenty-first century has been good for our Meadows.'

'Don't talk to me about that old rum-head! If job so plentiful, how de only one he get is to pick up tourist rubbish on de beach? What he know about these foreign devils? He have no education!'

Kat was fully aware of Mother Cynthy's distrust of foreigners. She knew her arguments and beliefs were set in concrete. Over the years they had all witnessed foreigners buying the most valuable lands of the Meadows and building huge brick hotels and plantation-style houses. Land people had lived on for decades, taken back by the government or bought from them for pittance and sold to foreigners for a fortune.

'The poor native can't afford to buy an acre in his own land no more, and when we work for foreigners they pay us peanuts, jus' like monkeys. A leopard can't change him spots and a white man can't change him greedy, oppressive ways.'

A stream of sweat sneaked down behind Kat's ears. She brushed it off with a flick.

'Miss Ruthie loves to boast about the Meadows. She says we have a better class of tourists than any other part of Jamaica. She says tourism is good for our country.' Kat's chin lifted with a challenge. 'It's the tourists who mostly buy my sketches and paintings. It's because of them I'm able to make a living, I can't be ungrateful for that.'

Mother Cynthy rolled her huge eyes until the whites showed and sighed heavily. 'Your mother finished school and marry your daddy all by sixteen years old. She and common sense are no relations.'

Kat chuckled but knew her own mother was right in one sense. People who came to the Meadows did not do so in search of a night life. They were neither young lovers out to experience pulsating love making on the beach, nor lager louts wanting their constant fill of alcohol. They were nearly always families with young children, anthropologists or archaeologists, spending their time in the numerous caves in the hills. On the other hand they were also the poets, painters and writers wanting the calm and tranquillity to complete a masterpiece. The middle-aged white ladies seeking young bucks were a recent addition and had come with the construction of a new hotel on the beach. Rumours had it that people walked around naked and had group sex in the sea, anywhere. She had heard the rumours but had never seen anything with her own eyes.

'I dream you last night.' Mother Cynthy's smile, like her eyes, courted mischief. 'Dream you were swimming with fishes. Let me see your hands.'

Mother Cynthy held out her plump ones, inviting Kat to do the same. Kat laughed lightly and raised her hands, palm up. Mother Cynthy peered quizzically.

'Ahh! It's here. See… It's here now! Look! Look!'

Kat looked at lined palms, which told no stories.

'Fishes in your palms! This can mean only one thing… one thing!' Mother Cynthy was clearly excited.

'I can't see any fishes, Mother Cynthy.'

'Yes, yes! Fishes, plain as daylight. I never wrong about these things. I wasn't wrong wid your mother and I not wrong now!' Her smile was soaked with satisfaction. 'But of course Miss Rootie won't like it. She going to be afraid for you but don't worry, it won't be easy but it won't kill you. I see complications with this man, though, he holds secrets,' she warned.

Kat could not stop her heart from leaping. Mother Cynthy was a wise soul and hardly ever wrong. The old woman dropped Kat's hands and stood up abruptly, looking frantically around.

'What is it, Mother Cynthy? What do you feel?'

'Someone watching you! I feel someone watching you!'

Kat looked towards the large crowd in the distance scattered along the beach front.

'There are so many people—'

'Yes,' Mother Cynthy cut her short, 'but only one watching with the eye of interest. Somebody watching you now! I feel it.'

Kat exploded with laughter, throwing her head back in excitement. Mother Cynthy had read her palm on her sixteenth birthday and had told her about a male figure, one from across the ocean that would steal her heart and make her a mother.

'So, the man you been telling me about, the one you

saw in my palm from across the sea, the one who will have a baby with me, he's here now?' Her voice dripped with tease but her heart hammered with hope.

Mother Cynthy was still looking around suspiciously. 'Uh huh! I feel him.'

Kat believed the old lady. She had to. For as far back as she could remember she had been warned that although she was able to, she shouldn't have a child. But she refused to believe it was in her best interest not to become a mother. Over the years Mother Cynthy's prediction had not paled in her mind, she was always reminded of it by the sight of a pregnant woman or a baby in arms. And now, Mother Cynthy was telling her her dream was about to come true.

Two

Thornton 'Ben' Benjamin

Jamaica

Since arriving in the Meadows, Thornton Benjamin had developed a fascination for the vast sea and its unpredictability. He felt no urge to venture into the waves and only really watched it as a scientist would watch an experiment—to discover something new. He appreciated the soothing breeze that skipped off the shore to brush his honey-coloured skin giving relief from the sweltering heat. His hair had been braided by one of the girls in the shops along the beach front, and she had given him eight tracks that ran down the back of his head, assuring him that he would be much cooler now. His eyes were hazel-green, depending how the sun shone and he had that chiselled jaw line that rendered him handsome by women's magazines.

Ben knew now why poets and writers loved to write about nature. It was the first time thoughts such as these roamed his mind and he put it all down to the romantic island of Jamaica. His mind had somehow developed an independent will and he could trace the origins of this new way of thinking to the first time he had seen the girl on the beach, comfortably sat on the flat rock, palm fronds shading her rich caramel skin, gazing out to sea.

He took his time strolling along the four-mile beach, the seeds of anticipation and excitement rambling in his gut at the thought of seeing her again and this time actually talking to her. He knew she would be sitting at the same spot under the palm trees looking out to sea or up at the sky. The sun was high above his head and the soaring heat sprouted beads of sweat on his forehead and laced his face with moisture.

A football landed on his chest jolting him out of his thoughts. A group of local children waved their arms, shouting, 'Hey, Mistah, kick back de ball.'

Ben kicked the ball back in the direction of the boys, missing them by a margin and making a group of screaming bikini-clad girls scatter instead. The small group of youths laughed as they approached him.

'Hey, Mistah, tek off your boots!' A lanky teenager, the tallest in the group and the obvious leader of the five gave him a friendly smile. 'You want us to teach you to kick ball? We can do it for twenty US. What's your name? People call me Dollar-Galore, but you can call me Galore.' He held out a long, bony, overconfident hand.

'I hope you'll make me pleased to meet you. I'm Ben.' Laughing he shook the outstretched hand. 'Can't stand around in this heat—'

'You hot? Want a drink? I'll take you to Rosie's Bar. Look!' Galore pointed ahead of them. 'It's that bar behind de fruit shop.'

Ben licked his lips as he encountered the crude structure of wood and zinc painted green, gold and black.

He smiled, nodding his head. 'How much will this cost me?' He had learnt that what typically cost the natives a dollar would cost him twenty.

Galore became animated, his long arm sliding around Ben's shoulders, steering him in the direction of the shack. 'Don't worry too much about that. A hundred US will do, nothing much cause you and me is bredren, friends.'

Ben humoured him. 'Yeah, bredrens don't charge each other one hundred US dollars for a bottle of drink! Do you think I'm crazy or what!'

'Okay. As you and me is good friends, give me fifty US,' Galore re-bargained.

Ben slowed his pace. 'How about I buy you and your boys a drink and a bun and we call it your lucky day?'

Galore rubbed his hairless chin giving the appearance of what he considered to be maturity.

'You and me is bredren, so I have to give you a good deal: drinks and buns and,' he lowered his voice, leaning towards Ben's ear, 'twenty US for me.'

'I don't have US dollars. I'm British, not American.'

'English! That's alright, just give me one of them pretty pink notes—de fifty ones.'

'Here's a fiver.' Ben thrust the note towards him.

'Thanks.' Dollar swiftly, discreetly and gratefully slipped the note into his pocket, glancing over his shoulder.

Rosie's open door shack wasn't much of a refuge from the searing heat. It was small and humid and no more than four people could fit comfortably inside. Most customers were local as Rosie's was an affordable day on the beach for them and they sat just outside on empty drink crates or near enough to stay shaded by the banana trees on each end of the small building.

'Rosie, set up my bredren Ben with five buns, four box juices and two Red Stripe,' Galore ordered.

Rosie sat in a wooden arm chair with a child clamped firmly between her thick thighs, weaving plaits into the girl's hair. She didn't look up until she had meticulously completed the task.

'Percy, how much time must I tell you that I am Miss Rosie to you. Have respect!' she stated without removing her eyes from her work. Rosie's skin was cinnamon with freckles sprinkled across her narrow nose and her full lips looked more appealing with a smile that revealed perfectly even white teeth. Her hair was in the long, neat plaits that he noticed the women and girls donned in the Meadows.

Ben looked at Galore with a smirk and mouthed, 'Percy?'

'My mother call mi that,' Galore said apologetically.

Rosie finally looked up, her eyes registering surprise when they met Ben's. She kept the comb moving through the little girl's hair, which had the child wincing with every stroke.

She smiled, taking in the man's handsome physique. 'Can I assist you, sir?'

Galore answered, 'Yes, you can. I tell you about de buns and de box juice and two Red Stripes.'

Rosie wrinkled her nose in distaste. 'You with him?' she asked Ben with wide disbelieving eyes.

'I'm just here to buy some drinks and get on my way.'

She pointed with her chin. 'Percy, help yourself and leave de money on de counter. I have to finish Tanisha's hair.' She smiled suggestively at Ben. 'You can come again another time when things not so hectic.'

He acted oblivious as he walked out, Galore and his crew closely behind.

'She wants some of you, man. She hot for you. Give me twenty English and I buy some of her for you.'

Ben turned the opposite way, ignoring the teenager. 'I have things to do now, so you guys enjoy your day. See you around.'

'We can flex with you, it's no problem,' Galore offered.

Ben turned to look at the group of boys. None of them older than sixteen and none with a decent pair of shoes on their feet. He felt a pang in his chest, remembering days where he looked not unlike them. He knew if he agreed to give them some money that he would become their source of income and nutrition for the day. Ben pushed his hand in the pocket of his shorts and pulled out Jamaican currency. He peeled a few notes and handed the majority to Galore.

'Buy you and the crew some decent trainers.'

The boys were transformed to eager puppies awaiting a treat. They circled Galore who stood transfixed, amazed at the wad of notes between his fingers. 'Thanks, sir, thanks and God bless you!'

The sun continued its assault as Ben walked on, taking periodic relief under the shelters of beach bars. Along the way one thought dominated his mind, the girl on the beach with the notepad. The sea-sky-gazer. He was a prisoner to his curiosity and the urge to meet her was as strong as the urge to sip an ice-packed glass of beer on a hot day. It had somehow become a challenge to approach her, which he admitted was ludicrous.

As he trekked to her end of the beach, he slowed his steps. The grains of sand found their way into his shoes and were sticking to his socks, but it did not matter, as there she was now sitting in front of him. As usual she was gazing out to sea and he approached her from behind, his shadow falling across her paper. She turned around suddenly, eyes wide and fired.

'Sorry, didn't mean to scare you,' he said quietly.

Her head jerked to where he stood and from her annoyed glare it was obvious she was reluctant to strike up any form of conversation. She relaxed back into a Buddha position, the sketch pad on her lap blank. He followed her eyes as they strolled from his shoe-clad feet to the top of his braided head. An amused smile softened her lips. He looked down at his shoes and thought that maybe they would seem strange to her. Suddenly her look of annoyance grew wings and sprouted curiosity.

'Are you from England, sir?' she asked in a soft Jamaican accent.

'Yes,' he replied, delighted she recognised he was English right away. 'My name's Thornton Benjamin but please don't ever call me Thornton, Ben will do.'

She laughed at the mock pain he pulled across his face and he noticed the small gap between the top two front teeth and the dark round pupils that left little space for the whites of her almond-shaped eyes, and the straight nose that flared at the tip. Her thick black hair was combed back and held by a brown clip into a ponytail.

'You should always wear white, it suits you.'

She looked down at her white cotton smock dress

then cocked her head to one side, observing him like you would something you were unsure, but not afraid of. He held her gaze for a few seconds and became even more alarmed by his own interest. He looked down, the round, tautness of her breasts beneath her dress briefly hypnotised him.

'You really love this spot. I see you here every afternoon with your sketch pad, looking out to sea, sitting so still and for so long... what are you looking for?'

Again she cocked her head as she looked at him. She seemed to be battling with a thought she was not prepared to share. Finally, hugging her knees she pierced him with her eyes.

'A Prince from across the sea, maybe. How I never see you watching me?' She looked intrigued and enchanted.

'You're always blue-skying.'

'Blue-skying?'

'Daydreaming... maybe about that prince from across the sea.'

A slow smile claimed her mouth. 'Blue-skying. I knew you came from England,' she boasted. 'There's four accents in this world that can't fool me. English, American, French and Italian. I know them well.'

'I'm impressed.'

'Are you?'

'Yes, that you're waiting for a prince from across the sea.'

He tried to read her eyes. Impossible. He was usually good at seeing through people's eyes but somehow she was managing to evade him. He surprised himself when he asked, 'How about lunch... sometime... maybe?'

Her silence was unsettling.

'I'm trying to get to know the place. It's my first time in Jamaica,' he quickly stammered.

'Obviously.' Her eyes lingered on his shoes.

He followed her stare to his feet again and thought of explaining, then changed his mind. How could he explain that he loved shoes? The lack of them in his early childhood meant he took the greatest pleasure in buying and wearing them now. He sat on the log facing her wondering what she would make of his shoe closet back home.

Ben broke the silence that had settled like a mist. 'People in Kingston said I could get some peace and tranquillity here.'

'Why do you need peace and tranquillity?'

He shrugged. 'Everyone does sometimes.' He sought her eyes again. Unreadable.

'So, what do you do? What's your name?' Ben asked.

'That's two questions from a stranger...'

'And you know what they say about strangers?'

'No, what?'

'They're friends you haven't met.'

'Strangers are friends you haven't met?' she repeated giving intense thought to the saying, savouring the words, tasting them like a chef would his cuisine. He watched her mesmerised. She remembered his questions. 'Let me see now. I'm an artist. I sketch, I paint, I teach and my mother has never forgiven me for throwing my English Catholic education down the drain. My name's Katherine St Monica Lewis, but call me Kat.'

'St Monica?'

'My mother is very, very religious.' Her voice sounded

musical, with an English vocabulary as the base and a Jamaican accent as the melody.

'You were schooled in England? At a Catholic school?'

'Catholic school, yes, but right here in Jamaica.'

'And you're an artist? You get paid to paint?' He was fascinated by this young woman and longed to learn more about her.

'Yes. I teach art classes too. I sell my paintings and sketches to the art centre, the craft market and local vendors. The tourists like them and I make an okay living. I have art exhibitions and auctions and I'm damn good.'

'Without a doubt. What do you paint?'

'Portraits, landscapes, anything.'

'If I commission you, will you paint me? Here at this spot?'

She looked into his eyes. He was amazed that human eyes could be so neutral. Yet there was something intriguing in them—a spark. As if big dreams danced unrestrained inside them. Layers, he decided. Her eyes were layered like the pages of a closed book. And with each turn of the page he discovered something new, different and mysterious. He would have liked to stay longer in Jamaica to try to understand her eyes.

'It could take a while.'

'I've got just two weeks,' he said with hope.

'I could sketch you,' she offered.

He smiled in agreement. 'Shall I meet you here, same time tomorrow?' he asked.

'Let me ask you something,' she said. 'Were you watching me yesterday?'

'I confess.' He smiled cheekily, raising his hands in

surrender. 'You and that character that walks like she's floating. I thought I was seeing a ghost.'

Kat exploded into laughter so big that it startled him.

'Mother Cynthy feels things,' she explained.

'What kind of things?'

Her voice held a deliberate tone of mystery. 'She feels some of what the future will bring.'

'Interesting. She must be rich, right?'

She laughed again. 'In spirit.'

'That's the best kind of wealth.'

'And what do you do? Are you here on holiday?'

'Now I am. I've been here two months working.'

'Two months! How I never see you before now?'

'I've been in Kingston overseeing a new build. Only paperwork left so I figured I'd finish it off by the sea. Folks said this was a great little off-the-beaten-track place to chill before heading home.'

'You're a builder?'

'No. I just love the strokes and curves of buildings. Got an eye for them, or so my boss tells me. I'm in real estate. I oversee projects to completion and then I market and sell them, taking my commission.'

'Is that enjoyable?'

He laughed at the astonishment on her face. 'Yes. It's hard work, but it's very rewarding, financially.'

She glanced at her watch. 'And finance is so important to enjoyment? You should know. Anyhow, I have to go now.'

He felt panicked and wanted to keep her talking longer. Was she offended by his talk of finance? He had to know. 'It's still so early—'

'It's a holiday for you but it's my everyday life. I have

to make a living so I'll meet you here tomorrow to begin your portrait, same time? Then eat afterwards.'

Disappointment washed over him. 'Okay. Money is important but not that important to enjoyment—' he knew he was babbling.

'No need to justify your preference. I'll see you here,' she smiled softly.

He grinned, relieved. Maybe she felt it too, this feeling between them. 'I'll see you tomorrow?'

She gazed at him, and he waited expectantly for the words that lay beneath the surface of her lips. But she seemed to change her mind and simply nodded, smiled and turned away. His feet felt glued to the sand as he watched her walk away, leaving behind an air of enchantment, entwined around him like ivy clinging to a pole. During that brief conversation something had been awakened in him, in his soul, a feeling heavy with danger yet so enticing.

Three
Miss Ruthie

6am as usual found Ruthie Lewis displaying fruits, vegetables and eggs on the long table in her front yard, ready for the first customer. Finally feeling satisfied with her display she climbed the wooden stairs onto her veranda and sat in her rocking chair, a basket of peas nestled on her lap. She meticulously picked out all the bad ones, throwing them to the chickens in the front yard. Periodically she dipped her hand into a brown paper bag on the small straw table to the side, taking a hand full of uncooked rice which she sucked, then crunched and swallowed. She hummed her favourite hymn, rocking to and fro as she continued shelling. The cry of the rusty hinges on the door made her look up.

'Good morning, Miss Ruthie,' Kat said, coming out of the house with a bag on her shoulder.

'Kat! Where you think you going at this time of morning? Sun hardly rise!'

'I have to see Poor George, you know I've been doing a portrait of his youngest grandchild and I've just got a few finishing touches.'

'The dew still on the ground! You want sickness take

you again, child?'

'Oh, Miss Ruthie, don't fuss. By the time I reach Poor George the sun will be hotter than hell and the dew gone. I'll see you later. Stop the worrying, no sickness will catch me today.'

'Is not the same day de leaf fall to the river bottom it rot!' Miss Ruthie wagged a finger. 'Let de sun gather some heat, Poor George can wait!'

'I made an appointment, it's business, he's paying me.'

Miss Ruthie breathed a heavy sigh. Ever since her daughter could walk, the child had done her own thing no matter how she cautioned. Kat's lips brushed her mother's cheek fondly.

'I'll be back in time for my evening meal, don't fret.' Kat took another glance at her mother. 'You looking very pretty, you expecting a visitor?'

Miss Ruthie ignored her last remark and presumptuous smile.

'And after Poor George I guess you going down to de beach to sit on that infernal stone and daydream about God knows what.'

'That's where my inspiration comes from. I'll be starting a portrait today of a Londoner I met yesterday so I may be a little late.'

'At least drink some bush tea before you go, 'member Mother Cynthy says it best to drink it first thing.'

'I had a cup already; in fact I had two. Satisfied?'

'Just because you don't get a sickle crisis in a couple years don't mean you cure,' warned Miss Ruthie.

Kat smiled tightly. 'And you need to always remind me about that, don't you?'

Miss Ruthie watched Kat disappear down the dusty lane which lead to the main road taxi park, her slim, athletic body moving with unconscious seduction and her mass of black hair bobbing in a ponytail behind her.

'I wish you was here to see your child, Glenrick.' Miss Ruthie wearily leaned back in the chair. 'She's a comely girl but she worry me with all her ambitiousness and strong will.'

Ruthie looked up a few seconds later to the scurrying of the chickens as the gate opened.

'Good Marning, Miss Rootie, talking to yourself again. The day look to be good and you look even brighter.'

Ruthie sucked on her teeth; the loud noise it created reflected her pretence at annoyance.

'Old Man, what you want to upset my day so soon?'

Her heart leapt. She silently cursed. It was too old to be acting like this.

'I'm here to wish you a good day, woman, and to buy a dozen limes and some eggs. You too pretty to give misery so many chances.'

Ruthie concealed her smile with a grunt.

'That pretty brown skin of yours and your Cooley hair so soft and plenty will make any man keep calling on you. Your eyes brown and enticing like brandy—I want to take you for a evening walk if only you agree. I want to start something good with you, woman.'

'You can start by walking your tired drunk old self out of my yard.'

'Oh Miss Rootie, I sober as a judge right now! Why you so stubborn? I calling on you year after year and you have not one kind word to give me.'

'We too old for that kind of nonsense. You with your rum soaked liver and me with stiff bones and a head full of grey hair. You think I want the whole Meadows laughing at me?'

Ruthie watched suspiciously as Old Man pulled up a worn stool and sat facing her. His cheeky old face looked as naughty as a teenager and she suddenly felt shy. She dipped her hands into the brown bag on the table and filled her mouth with rice. And her silly heart kept up its adolescent behaviour.

'My heartbeat is yours, Miss Rootie. I loved you from the moment I see you, even at your wedding. You were such a little girl when you married Glenrick.'

Ruthie's teeth crunched through the rice irately.

'I upset you now I can see it in your eyes but I telling de truth, and I wiser now, not playing games. I love you, Miss Rootie, I always have.'

She turned her eyes to the skies in a silent prayer, signing the cross. The barking of the dog momentarily distracted her.

'Stop that infernal barking, Samson.' The black Labrador ran to the back of the house, dispersing the flapping chickens.

Out of the corner of her eye, Ruthie could see her least favourite person stop by her gates, under the shade of the almond tree, as per the custom. 'Blessed morning, Miss Rootie,' the woman called out.

'The same to you, Nellie Potato,' Ruthie said to the post mistress, whose protruding stomach was the first thing anyone noticed before the darting devious eyes and loose lips, and who walked with a limp that the doctor supposedly diagnosed as an arthritic hip. She talked about it with such pride that you'd think it was some kind of lifetime achievement award.

'It look to be a good day, no rain in the sky or the air. I going to come in a while to pick up mi provisions, after I do mi Christian duty and take this breakfast to old Miss Bell.' She held up the basket in her hand. 'You going someplace important, Miss Rootie? You looking dressed.'

Ruthie blushed. Her hair was ironed and curled under her straw hat and her yellow cotton dress wasn't what she would usually wear mid-week. She looked at Nellie Potato with disapproval as a knowing smile touched Nellie's lips and her eyes danced from Ruthie to Old Man.

'Now you will have all de folks talking,' Ruthie muttered under her breath. She knew Nellie Potato disapproved of any woman over thirty who dressed up on any day other than Sundays. Especially a woman who had widow status.

'How is Kat? Not seen her in church lately or prayer meetings but she always down the beach mixing with the foreigners,' Nellie commented. She finally addressed the man beside Ruthie. 'Blessed morning to you, Old Man.'

Old Man dipped his head without uttering a sound. Nellie turned away without another word. Once Nellie had disappeared down the road, Ruthie adjusted herself in the chair.

'Did you hear her passing comment on my child for not going to church? I warn Kat all the time this would happen. Folks will talk if they don't see her face in church. They'll say she don't love God and Pastor

Green might hear.'

Old Man pulled a hand across his forehead wiping away the sweat. 'Pastor Green have plenty things to do, he don't have time for tripe.'

'And what you know? You don't go to church since Jesus was a baby.' Ruthie started picking the peas again. 'Kat should go more often because she get more sick. God forbid if anything happen to her, it would be Pastor Green perform the ceremony and him might not want to do it if she don't go church regular. I wish she would listen.'

'Leave Kat be, Miss Rootie. You know she don't care what folks think.'

'Well I don't hold with people gossiping, but it hurt me here, Old Man.' Ruthie patted her chest. 'It seems every year they be waiting for her to die from the sickle and for me to die from a broken heart soon after.'

'Folks are jealous of you, always have been. Don't mind them. You have plenty beauty. Just look on your smooth brown skin, there's no wrinkles on you! And your fine slim, womanly body. Nellie Potato fat and round like a pumpkin. I don't know how Farmer Tom get on top of her without rolling off.'

Ruthie grabbed a folded piece of paper and fanned her face frantically, swallowing the urge to laugh. It always gave her great pleasure when someone poked fun at Nellie Potato, which she admitted was not very Christian.

'You better leave now,' she told him. 'I won't be hearing your blasphemous talk. Your blood probably full of rum. Shoo now.'

'Miss Rootie, I swear one day I won't return and you'll

miss me!' Old Man wagged a finger before walking off.

Sadness welled inside her. Old Man Jaguar had been calling on her for many years, the words out of his mouth coated with sugar and sweeter than any cane. She held up a hand to call him before lowering it quickly, seeing Nellie Potato heading back her way.

*

Ruthie Lewis gave her husband Glenrick a child two months before her fortieth birthday. They married when she was sixteen and he twenty but no children came in all those years. As usual folks all had their reasons; Glenrick suffered with sickle cell anaemia and was in and out of hospital; his blood was bad so he couldn't have children. Ruthie sucked on raw rice as some children sucked their thumbs or fingers and others walked around with comfort blankets; or an even more far-fetched reason, *obeah*. Anything that could not be explained had to be *obeah*, witchcraft. If you were healthy and suddenly fell sick, it had to be *obeah*.

In those early days Ruthie's close friend, Cynthy, had started giving readings, a gift the town believed was handed down from her Maroon mother. Cynthy's predictions were becoming known as near to the truth as you could get. If she dreamt you, it was a sure thing that whatever she saw in that dream would befall you sooner or later.

'I see a baby girl, a wild child with a strong will and a stubborn streak,' Cynthy had foretold Ruthie.

'When she coming?' Ruthie was eager to know.

'I see no years, no time, just a wild child, a baby girl. Just trust the Lord, because as sure as the sun rise each morning, you will have that baby.'

'Cynthy says we going to have a baby girl, Glenrick.' Ruthie spoke to her husband's chest, his arms a comforting armour around her. She looked up to meet his silence. He frowned, his eyes piercing her, the pupils so large they nearly filled their entire socket.

Ruthie shifted guiltily. 'She read my palm and said we would get a baby girl.'

She felt him stiffen and quickly defended her action. 'I know how you feel 'bout that, but it wasn't *obeah*, it was just palm reading.'

'Oh Rootie girl, what I going to do with you? Don't waste good money on foolish predictions!'

'Cynthy never charges me a cent, Glenrick, and she's never wrong!'

When two months later Miss Ruthie discovered she was pregnant, her first port of call was to visit Cynthy, who was not surprised to see her. She smiled knowingly, her eyes tinged with sadness and a frown rested on her brow like a permanent scar.

'Tell me why you look so sad 'bout my good news?' Ruthie enthused.

'I happy for you, Miss Rootie, jus' 'member sey life is bitter-sweet. It gives and it takes.'

'Is it about the ashes you see me rolling in? Tell me, Cynthy, what it really mean? Is my baby in harm's way?'

'No. You will have your baby, a girl. These visions don't walk straight' was all Cynthy would say.

From that moment on Ruthie bestowed the title of 'Mother' on Cynthy and she became fearfully and respectfully known to the town folks as 'Mother Cynthy.'

Ruthie and Glenrick celebrated with a big party, inviting nearly the whole of the Christian town to celebrate with them. They were going to be parents at last. Glenrick finally received those congratulatory slaps on the back and shoulders, tobacco leaves, a Cuban cigar and bottles of rum and Ruthie could finally hold her head up among pregnant women. It didn't matter that most of her contemporaries were now grandmothers, she would be a mother and had proven the power of prayers and her belief in Mother Cynthy had paid off.

However, amid the clouds of happiness hovered uncertainty. Nine months later, Ruthie was taken to the main hospital twenty miles away where she gave birth to Katherine St Monica Lewis on a Monday afternoon, two minutes past one. Glenrick arrived with half the village who were refused entry. He looked so happy and so ill, Ruthie noted. She told him to take things easy while she was in hospital. She didn't like the yellow tinge to the whites of his eyes but she didn't want to dim the glow his new daughter brought to his face by pointing out such a thing. He was drunk with happiness at the sight of his baby girl.

'Look, Rootie, our own baby girl. We did it! The money in de bank, we going to send her to that Catholic school. The one where all the white children go. Our girl will have white teachas and speak good hinglish! She will be a lady.'

'Yes, praise the Lord! You taking care of you, Glenrick?'

'Oh, Rootie girl, don't fuss, I happy like lark!'

'But you looking like something coming on you. You

feeling sick? Go get some of Mother Cynthy's brew—I know you not into that but it won't do no harm to try.'

'Rootie girl, sickness couldn't touch me right now. I feel more joy than I can bear.' His smile filled the room.

'Is not the same day leaf fall to the river bottom it rots, Glenrick. You been burning the oil for too long. You simmer now.'

He smiled like a guilty school boy. 'I love you girl, always.'

He picked up his baby daughter and rocking her gently he whispered, 'Thank you Kat, for coming and please forgive your mama for calling you St Monica. You hearing me, baby girl? You listening to your daddy? I want you to give your mama plenty joy, make her laugh till she have to hold her belly. Make her proud and give her a grandson to run round her feet in her old age.'

Then he danced with the tiny baby in his arms, waltzing around the hospital room, a wonderful sight for Ruthie, the only sight that consoled her for the years that were to come.

Three days later she was still in hospital when she got the news that Glenrick was in the general intensive care unit. They wheeled her down to see him, but she knew it was too late. She didn't need to see his face to know his essence had gone. Glenrick Lewis was too alive to be that stillness fed by tubes on the railed hospital bed. She stood on shaky feet and whispered her farewell to the atmosphere where she felt his spirit lingered.

'Every goodbye ain't gone and every shut eye ain't sleep. Go with the Lord, my love, don't go holding on to suffering jus' for us.'

Then darkness with the hue of ashes enveloped her

like Mother Cynthy had foreseen, and she sunk to the cold, tiled hospital floor and wailed. One week after their daughter was born he was gone. Liver failure caused by his sickling blood cells. To add gun powder to the bonfire her tiny daughter was diagnosed with having the same disease that had afflicted her father his entire life. Sickle cell anaemia. Her first few months of life were spent in hospital and her prognosis was bleak. She wasn't expected to survive her first birthday. But, miracle has it, over the years, after every attack of sickling or infection that wrecked her young body that child would come bouncing back with even more life, passion and energy.

Four

Ben

Since meeting her, thoughts of Kat had not left Ben's head. Her smile, big laughter, and eyes gate-crashed his thoughts like a weapon, reducing his right-thinking to chaos. He made his way towards the spot with the flat rock and the palm trees, his heart leaping on catching sight of her. She saw him too and waved while talking on her mobile phone.

'I'll call you back later, Columbus. Yes, can't wait to see you too'. She finished her conversation as he neared: '*Au revoir.*' Her smile was warm as she waved the sketch pad and pencil. 'Hey, Ben, I've got my tools ready for you.'

It was like meeting an old friend. No need for nervousness or formality.

'Hey, you.' A smile curled his lips. 'I never knew you could speak French.'

'There's a lot to know about me.' Her smile was secretive. 'But I don't really speak much French, I just understand some of it.'

He joined her under the palm tree being careful to sit on the piece of log and not the flat stone throne she occupied like a queen. 'I see. You really going sketch me?'

Her brows arched teasingly. 'What else are you here for?'

He laughed, stroked by embarrassment.

'Don't put on shy with me,' she warned light-heartedly. 'There's no time for shyness. Life's too short and tomorrow's promised to no-one.'

'I hear you. Any reason for such a sombre proclamation?'

It occurred to him that despite the seemingly carefree and teasing manner there was seriousness and depth to her. Her eyes looked at him thoughtfully but again conveyed no clear message.

'I guess I want to live every moment like it's my last,' she finally said.

'Exhausting.'

They both laughed.

Kat clutched her notepad and smiled. 'Let's get started, I only have two weeks minus one day with you and I want to capture the spirit of you as I see you.'

He relaxed. Overhead brilliant blue skies, bluer than any blue he'd ever seen, stretched and disappeared into the lulling green sea. The sun was bright and hot but the cool breeze was a constant. Ben could easily believe that he was in another dimension. He sat quite still as his new friend sketched, her hand swiftly moving across the page as she traced him onto paper. Her eyes probed his face and she commented on the untidiness of his braids.

'I got it done on the beach last week,' he admitted ruefully. 'It needs re-doing. Can you braid?'

'Uhh uhh, when the feel take me.'

He laughed. 'You have a way of stringing your words together... I like it, it's very Jamaican.'

'It's a Meadows thing. Do you have a wife?' The question sprung out of the blue and dangled unanswered for a few seconds.

'No.' He had lived thirty-three years and thought he knew himself inside out but his response proved him wrong.

'Are you involved? You have a sweetheart?'

He continued to astonish and dismay himself by replying, 'No-one special.'

Kat laughed before continuing her work. 'Am I stirring the buried?'

'What?' He was starting to feel nervous about the lie he had just told. It was unlike him to lie, but he felt he needed to explore this budding relation with Kat. The truth would only complicate things.

'Are my questions digging too deep?'

'No, not at all,' he lied again, never having met a girl this direct before.

'You look at me like a new breed. You ever had a Jamaican girl?'

He laughed, marvelling at the contrast between his wife, Claire-Louise, and this free spirit. Claire-Louise would never be seen in public in anything less than her full face of make-up, her hair perfectly dressed, her toe and finger nails manicured, pedicured and matching, sprayed from head to foot with whatever latest designer scent she took to. Kat however was a breeze of her own. He sensed it. Her smooth caramel skin was devoid of make-up and her hair was simply tied in a bushy ponytail. She wore unfussy clothes; orange shorts and a white T-shirt with a slogan that perhaps said the most about her, *I Am Me*, and on her slender feet, pink flip-flops that had seen better days. He was wowed by her simplicity. She was fearless but he also sensed sobriety in her. And there was something else, that spark that he had noticed the previous day. Kat ignited his curiosity like no-one before.

'No.' That was true. 'Jamaican girls come with a warning in London,' he chuckled.

'A warning? What kind of warning?'

He laughed at her naked disapproval. 'Relax. It's a known fact that once you've had a Jamaican woman you want no other. They're good mothers, good home-makers and good lovers... some say.'

There was a hint of a smile before she changed the subject. 'You have any children?'

'Yes.' That he could not deny. They were his pride and joy.

'You are blessed, truly blessed,' she enthused, placing the pad on her lap and looking excited. 'Boys or girls?'

'Girls, two of them, India and Kenya.'

'Named after countries, whose idea was that?'

Her eager questioning was uncomfortable. 'Mine.'

'From the same mother?'

'Yes. Do you have any children?'

As her eyes swooped away from him he felt sure he caught the reflection of a mood, like a veil had slipped for a nano second.

'No.' She once more transferred her attention to the sketch pad. Her energy had changed and there was a sadness about her response that made him feel he had trespassed on private ground.

'Sorry.'

'For what?'

'I don't want to seem intrusive.'

'Being interested or curious isn't being intrusive.'

Her smile was soft and comfortable. An uneasy feeling filled him, drip by drip. During the last few hours he had changed his history, denied a big part of his life, wiped his wife out of existence. And for what? He wasn't sure. All he knew was Kat Lewis was the breeze which swept the boat he occupied out to sea with its hypnotic, seductive pull. He had no control over where the breeze would take him or if he would survive the journey. Yet he anticipated an exciting destination. Perplexity pulled him into silence. He was desperate to understand his feelings for her.

Her voice brought him back. 'I like your face. It's a kind face... a little too pretty for a man, but there's gentleness in you.'

'And you're very kind,' he responded automatically. 'Do you mind having lunch earlier? I missed breakfast and I'm hungry enough to eat a horse.'

She nodded and packed her materials away. 'I know the perfect place.' She stood to her feet rather stiffly, he noticed.

'You hurt your back or something?' He reached out to assist her.

She avoided his reach irritably.

'Sorry, Miss Independent or what!' He held up both his hands, only half-joking.

She smiled sadly. 'I'm sorry, I didn't mean to make you feel bad. It's just that I am capable of standing on my own.'

He slowed his pace to hers as they headed towards the taxi stand, her moment of frost confusing him. 'Who's Columbus?'

Kat seemed to ignore his question as they walked to Dutchie, a nearby restaurant. It was a rustic thatched roof building supported by four sturdy wooden beams. The tables and chairs were made of bamboo, the chairs mounted by soft hand-stitched cushions. Inside, it was dark and the air conditioner blew icy-cold, a welcome respite from the heavy heat outside. Colourful paintings of rural Jamaican life decorated the walls and a huge picture of Bob Marley with a lit marijuana joint hanging from his lips took centre stage. Reggae music played softly adding a mellow vibe. Ben pulled out a chair so that Kat could sit before he seated himself. She smiled from across the table.

'You were talking to him on the phone.' Ben eagerly resumed his previous conversation.

'Who?'

'Columbus.'

'Oh.' She seemed surprised Ben was mentioning his name. 'He's one of my best friends. He's French and adorable.'

Her eyes were downcast as she studied the menu so he couldn't read them.

'Adorable? Your best friend is a guy? A French guy? That's why you can speak French?'

'I don't really speak French...'

'Of course not, you just understand it.' He was aware how sarcastic he sounded but could do nothing about it.

'Uhh huh.' She continued reading.

'Interesting.' He picked up a menu and pretended to

read.

'What is?' Her tone carried no interest and she was still preoccupied.

'Your use of the term adorable.'

'He is adorable. He is a very good friend.'

'Most of the so-called platonic relationships I've known between men and women always, always end in bed.'

That made her look up from her menu and he folded his, anticipating a debate. Instead a superior smile crossed her lips.

'Most isn't all,' she said deftly, her eyes holding an invisible challenge.

Her response muted him. He had been preparing for a war of words, or a denial at the least. He'd never met anyone so unconcerned.

'How did you learn about this place?' he asked, looking around with new interest.

She answered, incredulous to his question, 'Everyone knows about Dutchie. It's authentic Jamaican food. Most tourists prefer it because it's the real McCoy, not like the hotels.'

Ben briefly glanced around at the filled tables. 'It's quite a busy place.'

'Anything authentic will attract. Now what shall we order?'

He left it for her to choose and she picked for him curried goat with rice and peas served with steamed vegetables. She ordered for herself brown stew fish, sliced and fried.

'You're spot on, this food is most probably the best I've tasted since I arrived.' He smiled with satisfaction, patting his stomach. 'A bit spicy though.'

'Your accent is so English, you act so English. You remind me of my English teacher Mr Bunting.'

'Ahhh! I forgot you're an expert on accents,' he laughed, reaching for his drink.

'Not only accents, mannerisms and personalities too.'

'Oh yeah?'

'You don't believe me? Take that group of tourists over there.' She signalled with her eyes. 'You don't need to hear them talk to know they're Americans, always ready to buy you a drink while telling you their life story. That group in the corner is definitely English. You can tell because they talk to each other very nice until they get drunk and then all hell will break loose, and they're mean. Italians over there.' She took a small sip of her juice. 'Beware of Italians. They smoke the most weed and will buy everyone a drink in the bar then tell the bartender they forgot their wallets at the hotel and will return. Only,' she giggled mischievously, 'they have a taxi booked to get them to the airport on the next flight out. And over there are the Germans, you can tell because they only talk among themselves, they don't mix. And that couple,' she pointed with her chin, 'French. They are the friendliest and the most romantic.'

'Are you talking from experience about the romantic French?' He was laughing, but also itching to know the real deal between her and this French guy.

'Yes. My friend Columbus is very romantic, but he is still only a friend.' Kat knew it wasn't going to be easy to explain her relationship with Columbus. It was complex and she could read the questions, the flickering doubts in Ben's eyes. 'Columbus and I have been friends for about ten years. Just friends.'

'Is that what he tells you or is it what you want to believe?'

'He has a thing for me I know that, but he doesn't cross boundaries.'

'I feel sorry for him,' Ben spoke calmly. 'I wouldn't want to be in your life for ten years and just be your friend.'

Their eyes locked over the calabash tumblers they were both sipping from. Neither said a word for a long minute but some aura flirting was taking place; invisible but very real. Kat was bubbling to tell Mother Cynthy that maybe, just maybe she had met the foreigner from across the ocean.

'But you're also my friend,' she pointed out teasingly.

'Not for ten years,' he laughed.

It could have been the ambience, the food or the rum punch but whatever it was, words came spilling from his lips like a cup overflowing. He started thinking about things that were so deeply buried inside that even he had forgotten how he felt about them.

'You remind me of this dream I had.' He couldn't believe he was really going to tell her about his recurring dream.

'What happened in the dream?' she asked, suddenly on the edge.

'I was relaxed, like I am feeling now. I knew who my parents were, at least my mother—' His voice broke. What was he doing? Telling her things that were so personal. Things he had shared only with his wife, Claire. There was this gaping hole inside of him. It was huge, but he had managed to effectively conceal it from the outside world. But now simply by her presence Kat had unlocked his vault of secrets and his tongue had no brakes.

'You mean you don't know your parents? Were you adopted?'

'My mother didn't want me. She abandoned me, left me for dead. For a long time I couldn't get my head around why a woman would give birth to a child then leave it outside a church wrapped only in newspaper never to return?' He shifted uncomfortably in his chair, his head twisting to ensure that no-one was listening. 'The social worker told me all they knew about me. And that was it. Abandoned outside a church in Thornton Heath and the police officer who found me was PC Benjamin—that's how I got my name. I don't even know my correct birth date; 25th October was just a guess made by those in authority.'

It had always been too painful to admit to anyone that no contact was ever made by his mother or relatives. No-one ever came forward to claim him and he had spent his life in grief, concealing the feeling of rejection and anonymity.

'Did you ever try to find her? Your mother?' Her voice was cautious but inquisitive.

'Thought about it. Thought about it a whole heap. Still think about it. But no. I was adopted by Professor Faintheart and his sister, Auntie Joan. She's the mother I never had. She lives with me now.'

'I don't think your mother was a woman,' she said thoughtfully, resting her jaw in her hand.

'What?'

'I think she must have been a very young girl, a

teenager too scared to tell her parents. She probably has never been able to forgive herself. But at least you're not bitter and after all you did get some care.'

The care system. He felt strongly about it being called 'care' because that was the least ingredient offered in the foster homes they farmed him out to. He couldn't bear to think about those dark, gloomy years filled with so much uncertainty. It got to the point that he would refuse to have his suitcase unpacked by the newest foster parent. Why should he bother? He knew it was only a matter of time before they got fed up and a social worker would arrive to move him to the next patch, until aged twelve, when he was no longer a boy but not quite a man, the Professor and Auntie Joan came along and adopted him.

His laugh was dry and humourless. 'When I had my children I learnt to forgive the person who left her baby outside a church. No-one in their right mind would leave a defenceless baby out in the freezing cold, she must have been out of her mind with some kind of grief or depression. Or maybe you're right, she may have been a silly, thoughtless, selfish teenager.'

He hadn't felt the tears leave his eyes in a trail down his cheeks. He didn't know they were tears until his tongue licked the side of his mouth and he tasted the saltiness. He suddenly felt self-conscious and held his head down in the hope that she had not seen his reaction.

'Or she simply didn't want an ugly baby, which no doubt you were. You're still ugly.'

He looked at her startled only to see the smile play around her mouth. He brushed the tears away laughing. He knew then she was intuitive. The moment needed lightness and she supplied it. She reached for his hand and squeezed his fingertips.

'Sorry.' He felt awkward as he responded to her touch. 'I usually don't do this... it's a first and last!'

'No need for sorry. Tears are human, you have feelings.'

Looking across the table at his friend of two days he felt overwhelmed, bewitched.

Back in his hotel room at Meadows Inn Ben paced, running his hand over his untidy braids. He was guilt-ridden at the comfort he felt with where he was heading. He buried his hands deep in his pockets and watched the waves crash against the cliffs time after time. Kat. He loved the working of her mind, the way she took her time to think before speaking. That melody in her voice. Her diction.

His mobile phone rang, interrupting his trance.

'Hi, Benny! I'm counting the days till you come home,' a female voice chirped on the line.

'Claire!' Ben exclaimed, pushing away all thoughts of Kat from his mind.

'Glad you remember your wife. It's always crazy trying to get through to you.'

'Hi, sweet girl, how are you? Where are the girls? Let me talk to them.'

'They're sleeping, remember the time difference is like six hours; it's after 4am here. I miss you.' Her voice was soft and pleading and pulled at his guilt.

'Me too. Everything okay? How did that charity event you helped to plan go?'

'It could have gone better if they'd taken my advice and invited the mayor, we would've raised more money for the Lupus charity... and of course Auntie Joan is always on hand to correct my every move.'

Ben chuckled. 'You know by now she means no harm.'

'I know you believe that! But even after all these years I feel she still disapproves of me. It's obvious to everyone but you.'

'Who's everyone? Auntie Joan is the salt of the earth and she loves you.' Ben was not going to take seriously any complaints against his mother figure.

'We could disagree all night on that subject'. A heavy sigh came through the phone. 'Can't you come home now? Bring your flight forward?'

Yes he could, but he wouldn't. He needed answers, needed to understand his actions, these new thoughts and even to get to know the person that stared back from the mirror. Because up until he met Katherine St Monica Lewis, he had thought he knew all he would ever know about himself. Now his curiosity had been stirred.

'In less than two weeks I'm home.'

'It still seems long. The girls are missing you so much, especially Kenya, and India is so moody, I'm sure she's going to start menstruating soon.'

Ben panicked. 'Rubbish! I've only been gone two months and she's only eleven.'

Claire chuckled. 'Benny, a lot can happen to a young girl's body in two months. And if I remember right, I think I was around eleven or twelve when I started.'

'But that was so long ago, don't things change?' He was concerned.

Her laughter softened his edginess. 'Your girls are

47

going to grow into women no matter what you think or how you try to baby them.'

'It's-it's just too soon, I mean she hasn't even got breasts yet—'

'Yes she has, she's a 30A in bra size.'

'Whatever that means, she hasn't got breasts, that's puppy fat.'

Claire's laughter was loud and he imagined her on the bed kicking her feet in the air, a thing she did when gripped by humour. 'Please do not let our daughter hear you say that, there's not an ounce of fat on her. Get accustomed, Daddy, in fifteen months or so we're going to have a teenager on our hands.'

Ben heaved. 'I miss you, and I miss my girls. Less than two weeks and the project will be over, I'll be all yours.'

'Good. Buy me a bag in duty free and some perfume, the latest DK will do.'

'Haven't you got enough bags and perfumes?'

'A girl can never have enough bags or perfumes.'

Ben flopped onto the bed looking up at the white patterned ceiling. That was the first time he had lied to his wife so blatantly. He didn't consider himself a Casanova despite the good looks people told him he possessed. He had no desire to bed all females who came within ten yards of him, much to the disappointment and disgust of his best friend, Bubs. His abandonment had always ensured he was firmly rooted in reality.

He looked in the mirror. His braids needed re-doing, perhaps Kat could do it? He shook his head. How had this happened? Something about her was magnetic, and he could not control his reaction, he told himself. Yet he couldn't deny his surprise at what he had revealed to her. Never before had he discussed his past so freely because of the hopelessness it stirred. But he had sat in a restaurant and poured out his soul to someone he had met forty-eight hours earlier and was mystified by it. His life had been turned around by Professor Faintheart and Auntie Joan. He knew about love and learned about morals and virtues, family values and loyalty. Now here he was deliciously poised at the edge of betrayal, but to his utter dismay he felt, if she said the word, he could not resist Kat.

Five

Ben

Ben woke early the next morning but stayed in bed mired deep in thought. The sun must have sensed his sombre mood because it too took time to light the skies. He reached for the remote control that turned on the air conditioner. The uneasy feeling that lingered in the pit of his stomach had its origin in Kat. He felt he should tell her about Claire so that there would be no illusion and she was clear about his position and what could and could not happen between them. He took deep breaths as the thought of Kat caused his stomach turbulence. She intrigued him. She enchanted him, causing him to count in hours, minutes and even seconds until he saw her again.

They met at two in the afternoon at the usual spot on the beach. She was first to arrive, sitting in her customary Buddha position, pad on her lap and pencil peeking from behind her ear. She waved as he approached and he waved back, his feet and heartbeat speeding up in anticipation he had yet to understand.

'Hi,' she smiled.

'Hey, you.'

She stood up, surprising him. 'I want to show you something amazing—want to see?'

'Sure.'

She started walking towards the road. He could not help but follow her, bewitched.

'It's a taxi ride as far as a car can go, then we have to walk the rest of the way. Can you manage the walk in those shoes?'

'I can run a marathon in them,' he retorted jokingly.

He tried to find out their destination, but she refused to reveal it, arguing the surprise would be worth the wait. Following behind her along the narrow dirt road, his nose teased by the fresh scent of the thick bushes and his fear heightened by thoughts of what could emerge from the forestry; he breathed a sigh of relief when they came to the bottom of the hill.

'This is the easy way up,' she told him, pointing. 'It has stone steps.'

She took him to the top of Meadow View, where the breeze was cool as they stood viewing the town below. The jade sea with its many speeding boats leaving their white water trail behind them made a beautiful picture postcard image. They were surrounded by baby's breaths, their cloud-like white heads and delicate stalks swooning with the persuasion of the breeze.

'Where are we?' he asked as he watched the scene from behind her.

'This is the Nyahbinghi Camp, some of the Rastafarians have created a community here where they live in peace, love and unity. Follow me, let's go see them.'

Soon they were sat around the blazing, leaping fire in the large compound in a circle of bearded dreadlocked men who were chanting in deep melodious tones, words that were slurred with emotion. The women, heads wrapped with colourful cloths, were separated from the men by the dancing flames. Older women held the Bible to their chest as they sang, young mothers had babies or toddlers cushioned in their arms, rocking to the shouts of the drums. Kat sat beside Ben, hypnotised by the sounds. He watched her, mesmerised by her complete focus, the serenity that gently enveloped her.

'Where are you?'

Without moving she answered, 'I'm travelling on a star.'

He chuckled.

She turned to view him with unreadable eyes. 'Don't you ever think what it would be like to travel to outer universes in your mind's eye?' Her voice was incredulous.

'No.' He wished his response had been different because the look that quickly swept across her face made him feel inadequate.

'I've got heaps to teach you.'

He caught something in her voice that sobered him immediately.

'Teach me!' he exclaimed indignantly.

She laughed and her eyes danced, laughing at him. It was the first time they had displayed such clear emotion.

'Don't be vexed. There's so little time,' she coaxed.

'Well, it's just that I've never thought about outer universes in those terms and I don't have friends who do either.'

'No, I don't suppose you do.' Laughter lingered in her voice.

They stayed in place until the bright blue afternoon

sun-soaked skies gave way to the deep orange and purple evening sunset. The view from that height was breathtaking and Ben could not help himself. He got his camera out and took photographs, as at the horizon the sun set its orange-red halo disappearing into the sea.

'Isn't nature beautiful?'

'Magnificent.' In all his travels he had never bothered with such things as watching a sunset.

'Don't you ever wonder how it never forgets to rise or set? The sun?'

'No, but I'm getting use to the fact that maybe I should?' he finished with caution.

Kat's laughter flaunted an invite for him to join in and he did. 'You should take some pictures of the baby's breath,' she said.

'The what?'

'Those flowers,' she pointed. 'Columbus brought the seeds back from Europe years ago and we planted them here. Just look at them now.'

'Baby's breath? I wonder why they called it that. Do you and Columbus often do things like that?'

'Like what?'

'Plant flowers together?'

Her smile was dismissive and he knew he would get no answer. He had already learnt that she did not respond to what she considered trivial, as if time was far too precious to waste on such things. He liked that about her.

'I love them. Doesn't the name baby's breath just say soft and beautiful? They're my favourite flowers.'

'Mine too.' He smiled mischievously.

She looked at him dubiously, then laughed at his

blatant lie.

'Miss Kat, nice to see you up here,' a voice called out.

The couple turned around to see an old man walking towards them.

'Ras Solomon!' she exclaimed, jumping to her feet and throwing her arms around the elder who embraced her warmly. 'Is Rosie here?'

'Yes, she just went to pick up a soup. Look at you!' He held her at arm's length and admired her from head to toe. 'You looking like something really sweet you.' His eyes twinkled as he looked towards Ben. 'Love agrees with you!'

'This is Ben, a friend,' she quickly corrected.

Ras Solomon held out a hand, dry and cracked from hard work. Ben shook it with a smile.

'Where you hail from?' Ras Solomon's voice was coarse as though it travelled over sand paper before it emerged from his mouth, and the whites of his worn and guarded eyes were tinged by red.

'London,' Ben told him.

'Babylon! The bridge still burning down?' He laughed at his own joke, a deep laugh that rattled. 'I was in Babylon in de sixties with me first wife, Babsy. I never like it—the place too cold and wet. Wet every minute and Babsy turn miserable. Life wasn't easy in the land they say paved with gold. It was more paved with the black man's blood and sweat!'

'White men's too,' Ben found himself saying. Ras Solomon looked at him like he would a mad man.

'You is one of them!' Ras Solomon expression was one of scorn.

Ben resented his look. 'All I'm saying is the Irish had

54

their fair share of shit too. It wasn't only black people who suffered; if you were poor you suffered too.'

'The Irish take care of themselves, we should take care of our own and stop letting the white man use us like tools. Of course poor whites suffer, but not as much as the poor blacks. Every race has used the black.'

Ben nodded in agreement. 'Yes, that could be true, I'm not disputing it. All I was trying to say is every race at some time experience injustice and sometimes what we do to each other as humans... well, it baffles the most intelligent minds.'

Ras Soloman shook his head gravely. 'You speak too generic, you study too long in the white man schools. He's brain-washed you, turn you in a fool!'

Ben laughed, hoping to dilute the heavy mood created by Ras Solomon's comments.

'England has a terrible history in the Caribbean. It built a lot of its fortune on the back of slavery but things and time have changed. It's a beautiful country, especially in the spring and autumn. London happens to be one of my favourite cities, and not just because I was born there.'

'I never find no beauty in Babylon. The white people use to put up signs in a window—no blacks or dawgs!'

'That's all changed,' Ben told him. 'On the surface at least. There are laws, now it would be illegal to put up a sign like that.'

Solomon was unconvinced. 'Laws can't change beliefs, all laws can do is send beliefs underground, make people more hypocritical.'

Ben nodded. 'I understand but it's a human thing that transcends the colour of your skin. Humans can do the most terrible things to each other. In the end it's about power, not just colour.'

Ras Solomon looked dubious; his hand thoughtfully stroked his matted beard. 'Power, yes, that is very important to the white man, but believe me, it's about colour too. Look how they set up their system: white is alright, brown can stick around, but black? Stay back! It's that simple! Everything black is negative.'

Ben looked at Kat who was so obviously enjoying the discourse and was eagerly awaiting his response.

'But do you know,' he argued, turning to Ras Solomon, 'that the most bought cars are black and they're also more expensive than any other colour cars?'

The rattle of Ras Solomon's laugh exploded from his opened mouth. 'You wise.' He grabbed Ben by the hand and shook it vigorously. 'I like a wise man.'

Ben found himself feeling honoured by the new gleam of respect that flickered in Ras Solomon's faded brown eyes as the elder shook his hand again before walking over to join the drum-beating men. Ben felt a warmth at being accepted by Kat's friend, as if he had passed a first hurdle. He stood smiling for a few seconds before the woman from the Shack, Rosie, appeared sipping from a steaming cup of soup.

'Hey, skinny girl, what you doing so far from home...' Rosie trailed off as her eyes picked up Ben. She raised her eyebrows at Kat.

'Oh, sorry,' Kat said. 'Rosie, this is Ben, and Ben, this is my good friend, Rosie.'

'We've met,' Rosie said, smiling sweetly at Ben. At Kat's puzzled look, she explained, 'He stopped by the Shack with Percy and his crew the other day. He bought them new trainers, Percy tells me.' She leaned conspiratorially towards Kat and whispered, 'You beat me. I was hoping to get my hands on candy eyes.'

Kat pushed her jokingly. 'I'll catch you later, Rosie.' She took Ben's hand and started pulling him away. 'Come. It's a journey down to town; we'll take the dirt road and pick up a ride along the way.'

By the time they got out of the back of the old Toyota truck at the foot of the hill, the moon was a white orb in the black velvet sky. Stars paraded decoratively, enticing and inviting the eyes to worship and adore them. They stopped off at one of the street vendors to purchase a cup of red pea soup, which Kat insisted Ben tasted.

'You like it?' she asked after he took his first sip.

'Very nice. It's very spicy and taste a little coconut-ish.'

'That's because it's made with coconut milk. It's very good for you and a little pepper won't kill you. You should have a cup a day. Ras Solomon is a chef, soup is the only cooked thing he lets pass his lips and he's nearly seventy years old!'

'Seventy!' Ben mocked surprise. 'He looks nearer sixty-nine!'

She laughed, giving him a friendly push. 'You held your own against him. Not many can, he likes you. He's a great person to know. Some say he has powers too. He feels things.'

Ben smiled. 'Another one! You have some strange friends. A Frenchman, a floating herb woman, a Rastaman and a man-eater! That Rosie is something else.'

She shrugged, laughing. 'Some say I'm a strange girl.'

They walked slowly savouring the night's beauty. They held hands as if it was the most natural thing in the world to do. Taxis passed them along the road, hooting their horns trying to pick up a fare. Ben waved them on and enjoyed the half-hour walk back to the town centre, serenaded by the songs of a thousand tiny insects.

'I'll take the taxi from here,' she told him, letting go of his hand. 'Miss Ruthie will be flapping like a bee in a bottle wondering where I am'.

'Who's Miss Ruthie?' asked Ben, desperate to make the moment between them last.

'My mother.'

'You call your mother, Miss Ruthie?'

She laughed. 'Yes. Everyone calls her Miss Ruthie.'

'What about your father?'

'He died when I was a baby,' she explained simply.

Ben shifted awkwardly, hoping he did not touch a sensitive spot. He cleared his throat. 'And you live with... Miss Ruthie?'

She nodded. 'She'll be sitting on the veranda with the oil lamp until I return. Won't move an inch till then.'

'It's early evening and you're a grown woman,' argued Ben.

'I've been telling Miss Ruthie that for years.'

Ben wanted not another minute to pass without telling her about Claire. The uneasy feeling wouldn't vanish until he did. The day had presented no opportunity and now she seemed in a hurry to get home.

'I thought maybe we could have dinner at a restaurant along the beach front. Can I tempt you with good conversation and philosophical logic? What about: Angels, do they exist? Or can dreams really come true?

Or is there life after death? Or where do the stars go during the day?' he suggested, hoping they would be able to talk privately.

Kat laughed. 'Not tonight. But angels do exist, dreams come true all the time and there is life after death. As for the stars...' She looked up to the sky. 'They don't go nowhere, they just change light so you can't see them in the daytime, but they are there.' She smiled before starting to walk away. 'See you tomorrow! I'll take you to the river. And wear sandals; give the shoes and socks a break!'

Ben chuckled, shaking his head as he watched her slow and enticing walk, responding to the greetings of people she knew along the way. He was still standing watching her when she eventually turned and waved at him. What was it that made her so calmly confident and nonchalant? He was completely smitten.

Six

Kat

If you've never observed limits, then anything and everything is possible. And that's how Kat saw life. Limitless. And every moment meaningful. Every meeting life-defining. She couldn't afford to see it any other way, and not the way that the folks in the Meadows, including her own mother liked to view it.

She sat in Miss Ruthie's rocking chair on the veranda, watching her mother serving and talking to the early morning customers. She felt warm inside, thinking of the day she had spent with Ben, the stranger from overseas. She looked at her watch, keeping an eye on the time because she was meeting with Paula, a childhood friend who was back on the island for the first time in ten years. Still she could not help thinking about Ben, whom she would meet after.

The joy this anticipation gave her couldn't stop the smile exploding onto her face whenever she thought about him. Ben. The prediction, the possibilities. She knew her obsession with having a baby was not most young women's dream, but then most women hadn't had the wish to have a child frowned upon by a whole town. It was made all the more frustrating because her internet research down at the library had turned up women from all over the world who suffered with the sickle, and had children without losing their lives. When she had pointed this out to Miss Ruthie, it just made her mad, so mad she began speaking in 'tongues.' When she had calmed herself, she sat Kat firmly down and reminded her how her aunt Doris, her father's younger sister, had died trying to give birth.

'And your Aunt Doris was a stronger woman than you. The sickle didn't take her as bad as it takes you, and having a baby killed her. If your father were here today he could tell you with his own mouth, you just forget about ever having a baby, you hear. Puss and dwag don't have the same luck.'

And that was always that with Miss Ruthie.

Meeting Ben and him admitting to watching her, just like Mother Cynthy felt on the beach the other day, was all too divine just to be a coincidence. She did house doubts about Ben, a foreigner, a handsome, obviously wealthy foreigner having an interest in her, a simple country girl. She couldn't help wondering why. With looks like his he could have his pick of any girl on the island, but he had chosen her to spend his two weeks in the Meadows with. He enjoyed her company. She liked that he seemed to appreciate her humour and frankness. She liked the way he looked at her too. The way his eyes smiled, that little way he had of holding her gaze as if trying to peer into her soul.

She startled, suddenly remembering where she was. She glimpsed at her watch, noticing how much time had passed and grabbed her bag from off the table.

Miss Ruthie looked at her enquiringly. 'Where you off to so early again?'

'I told you, Paula is back in the Meadows, I'm going to see her and my marvellous goddaughter.'

'Mrs Smith daughter, Paula? Didn't she marry a African man? Broke her father's heart her going to the other side of the world with people we don't know.'

Kat looked at her mother wearily. 'Miss Ruthie, what's that supposed to mean, "with people we don't know?" Paula knew him and that's all that matters in today's world, don't you notice?'

Miss Ruthie pursed her lips defiantly. 'Those Africans worship different things. They have chiefs they listen to and revere and witches too. It all sounds very pagan, very suspect to me. Our Lord Jesus would not approve.'

'And you listen to the pastors and revere their words, which sounds suspect to me.'

Miss Ruthie ignored her daughter's comment. She snatched the broom that was leaning against the table and occupied herself as Kat smiled secretly and went on her journey.

Paula hadn't changed, Kat observed as they sat under the palm trees that shaded the strip of beach in front of Hotel Panama. Entrenched in the air, the smell of alcohol, smoking jerk chicken and baked fish. Paula's dark chocolate skin was unblemished and untouched by the years, and her afro was still the same after all these years. They sat sipping coconut rum punch on glass designer sunbeds that had spongy gold velvet cushions, keeping a close eye on Paula's two children, Sian and Ella who were playing with a ball and plastic bats. Cradled in

Kat's arms was the newest edition to Paula's family, her three-month-old son, Wesley.

'Paula, you are so lucky,' marvelled Kat who brushed her nose over the fine downy hair on the baby's head, inhaling noisily. 'I just love the smell of babies, there's nothing like it in the world.'

'They don't smell like that all the time.' Paula smiled, reaching out to stroke her baby's cheek. She focused back on Kat with a grin, eager to hear all the local gossips. 'So tell me, what's been going on in sleepy Meadows these last ten years?'

'Nothing as exciting as Namibia, I'm sure,' Kat said pointedly. 'You know most people in the Meadows still can't pronounce Namibia, their tongues get twisted so they just say Africa.'

Paula laughed. 'It was like that for me at first too.'

Baby Wesley stirred and Kat held her breath; he was so small and she was conscious of being careful to the point of stillness.

'You can relax,' Paula told her, 'babies can feel tension, sit back and just breathe, he'll be fine.'

Kat released her breath with a laugh. 'Was it so obvious? He's so tiny, Paula. Is Robert happy with his son?' she asked, thinking of Paula's husband.

'Ecstatic! You know how men in general are about sons, but African men are very, very proud. He adores his daughters but he's smitten by his son. And of course I get points with his family for having a boy.' She rolled her eyes and shook her head. 'This cultural shift toward boys drives me crazy, Kat.'

'You must be so proud of yourself, Paula. You're my hero.'

Paula laughed, amazed. 'Me? Are you crazy? What have I ever done other than getting pregnant out of wedlock and causing shame and scandal on my family?'

They both laughed and Kat was reminded of why she and Paula had become friends in the first place. Paula had been a challenge to everything and everyone during their childhood, and in some sense more the talk of the Meadows than Kat. She was an extremely exceptional student who won a bursary to study Math in America when she was eighteen. When she was twenty, news broke around the Meadows that Paula had messed up her opportunity in America and was having a baby with an African man she had met at university, and that he was taking her away to his country to marry her or worse, kill her.

'I got lectured for months and months after news broke about you being pregnant. Miss Ruthie didn't miss a chance to mention how you broke your poor mother's heart and nearly killed your daddy.'

Paula shook her head. 'People are so backwards, how do you manage to still live here, Kat? I always thought you'd be one of the first to leave the Meadows. You were always day-dreaming looking out to sea, as though something was calling your soul. I remember you could be still for hours. We'd leave you on the shore while we went to swim and when we returned, it's like you never moved. And you didn't care what people thought about you, about you having "sick blood" as the fools call it. I mean sickle cell anaemia is not contagious, but these idiots—' Paula heaved.

'They still have those beliefs and you can't tell them different,' finished Kat, shaking her head.

'You need to leave the Meadows, Kat. Take your art further, you're so talented, the world should know your gift. Also, find yourself a good man and have a family. Is there a Mr someone-special lingering?' Paula teased.

Kat hesitated for a few moments but finally decided to confess her interest in the gorgeous stranger to her friend. 'I met someone recently. He's from London.'

Paula straightened up. 'London? You thinking of moving to London? That's a smart move.'

Kat shook her head smiling. 'I've only just met him! Remember when I phoned you and told you about Mother Cynthy's prediction?'

'Ummm, that's a long time ago,' Paula recalled. 'That you're going to have a baby with someone from across the sea or something.'

'Yes. Well I think this could be him. Ben. He's nice. Or seems.'

'He's the one you're going to have the baby with?'

Kat nodded, willing to believe Mother Cynthy's prediction. She had never been wrong before, no matter what other folks said.

'So how will it work? You're going to get pregnant for him deliberately?' Paula asked dubiously. She waved a hand to her daughters, beckoning them to come closer. 'Is he going to know about this prediction?'

'He will if it's fate, Paula,' assured Kat.

Her friend shook her head. 'We influence our own fate, Kat, that's what I've come to believe.'

'And I think we have no control over fate or destiny, that's beyond us. I don't really know anything other than what Mother Cynthy said. But if she sees me having a baby then it means I won't die, that I can be a mother.'

'Of course you can. All that gibberish them old people like to pass on to us is only that, gibberish. It's the same in Nam, so much cultural superstitious stuff. Pregnant women don't die from sickle anymore, only if maybe they have other complications.'

'I know, Paula, I've tried telling Miss Ruthie but she won't hear it. She just wants to remind me of Aunt Doris. Then of course I get a bit doubtful and scared because the reality is that she did die giving birth and her sickle crises were not as bad or as regular as mine.'

'Puss and dawg don't have di same luck!' Paula mimicked in Miss Ruthie's voice and Kat laughed. 'Anyway,' Paula continued, 'how's Rosie, how many kids now? And how's your Frenchman, Columbus?'

'Rosie's stopped at number five, she says and Col is back in Paris with his mother, taking up his role as VP in her perfume company and then he'll go spend time with his father in Scotland.'

'How the other half lives,' Paula smiled enviously. 'What I'd give to be a VP in my family's business and get to roam the world for six months of the year. You know that's a white male privileged thing, right?'

'Col would disagree. He would tell you how hard it's been going against the plans his parents have for him, and being the only child of acrimoniously divorced parents who use him as a pawn in their battle. He's had to be strong to follow his own passion. He loves to travel and he loves the Meadows.'

'And when will Kat take a trip across the ocean, come visit me in Nam? It would be lovely to have you stay for a while, see another part of the world.

And you could come and explore other possibilities outside of the Meadows.'

Kat looked thoughtful. 'Maybe one day.'

Seven

Ben

Kat sat on her throne the following afternoon, sketch pad and pencils ready. The sea was riotous and crashed against the rocks, its fine white froth carried by the breeze sprayed them. Ben licked his lips, tasting the salt the spray from the sea deposited, and smelling the raw fishy odour from the ocean's life. It was another busy day on the beach, and from where he sat he could see the holiday makers playing volley ball and table tennis, girls in skimpy bikinis and the men, bare chested and showy. Then right next to all of that, sun beds lined up with the bodies of differing shapes and sizes, basking in the hazy glow and being served ice cold beverages on trays from the beach bar waiters and waitresses. The coconut and palm tree lined beach looked idyllic and it was easy to see why people would work their butts off and save a whole year to experience even just a week of this tropical dream.

Kat could not know that Ben had another uneasy night that had left him feeling reflective and irritable. She was not to know that he needed to unload the truth about himself, his marriage, because it was grating against his insides. Yet he was fearful of telling her—the thought that she might not want to see him again was ridiculously unsettling.

'A choppy sea means there's rough times ahead and a warning that great courage will be needed,' she warned, teasing. Her hair was tied in two plaits that rested on her shoulders, held together by yellow elastic bands at the ends. She looked young, more like a girl of eighteen than a woman of twenty-eight.

'Does everything have to mean something to you? Can't the sea be rough because of climatic changes?' he snapped, feeling her comment hit too close to home. He immediately regretted his words as disapproval coloured her face. It was still a puzzle to him how she kept her eyes so clear of feelings, an act he guessed must have taken many years of practice to accomplish.

'You are a real doubter, Thornton Benjamin. Why can't everything have a meaning? Would that be so bad?' replied Kat, frowning.

'Not bad, just unrealistic because there are more questions than answers.'

'I agree, some questions have to go unanswered, but it doesn't mean there's no answer for them.'

Once again, she managed to make him doubt his life-long convictions with one simple but thoughtful comment. His best friend Bubs had on many occasions tried to alter his thinking, his character, but failed miserably. He was his own man and would never allow anyone the privilege of tampering with his personality, his beliefs or his principles. But Kat was different. She had the knack of saying things that made complete sense and which required no questioning. He reluctantly admired this about her.

Kat began to sketch. 'What are you considering so hard today?' she asked. 'Don't tell me you let Ras Solomon get under your skin after all!'

'I actually liked Ras Solomon. He has strong opinions but that just strengthens his character. No, it's not him. It's me. I need to explain something.'

Kat raised her head, detecting his discomfort. 'Only if you want to.'

'I do,' he grimaced, feeling he could not put off this difficult conversation any longer.

Putting the pad and pencil down, she turned her full attention on him. Once again, he could not read her.

'How do you make your eyes do that?' he asked with wonder.

'What?'

'Be so inexpressive. Usually I'm good at reading peoples' eyes, but I cannot read you at all.'

Her laughter soaked the air around him, massaging his nervousness away. He decided he also liked her ability to make a mole hill out of a mountain and to convince you of the same.

'Tell me what you need to explain and don't beat about the bush, there's such little time for us. In a little less than a week and a half you'll be back in your world and it will be like we never existed to each other.'

Her words struck him dumb. Less than a week she'd be a memory. The idea was unbearable and preposterous. She was right; they should just enjoy their time together. He was four thousand miles from home seduced by sun, sea, sand and opportunity. Nothing untoward had happened between them, they were just two adults enjoying each other's company. Perhaps he needed to spend time with her to explore who he really was outside of his little world.

'I want you to know that I really appreciate you spending time doing my portrait,' he finally said. It sounded lame even to his own ears and he knew she would question it.

'That's it?' She threw a dubious look at him.

He nodded, feeling even more uneasy.

'Don't look so fretful,' she told him. 'I never squeeze the tail of a dog to see if it's sleeping.'

'What's that supposed to mean?'

'I'll mind my own business. You obviously don't want to tell me what's really playing your mind.'

Ben laughed nervously. 'What do you think you could stir?'

She shrugged her slender shoulders. 'Everyone has something to stir.'

'I can't help feeling that you hold things inside that most people would never understand. What's your secret? I command you to reveal it,' he teased.

He had expected her to erupt in her usual laughter; head flung back, hand on heart. She barely smiled. Her eyes misted and he waited to see what feeling would be reflected. But as the mist cleared they remained unreadable. She was closed again, like a clenched fist.

'What have I said? When you look at me like that I feel like an idiot. What fundamentals did I miss this time? I really want to understand.'

She suddenly reached for her cloth bag and put her sketch pad and pencils in.

'You missed nothing. It's so hot. No sketching today. You want that river bath now? It will cool us.'

They hopped in a taxi to Rising River, where the sea meets the river deep in the mossy green valley of the Meadows. The taxi meandered along the narrow road, the driver avoiding potholes with skilful sways. Ben looked out of the window and realised that one wrong move would usher the car over a precipice. Kat chatted with ease, telling him of her love for the river and how peaceful the place was. He half listened, keeping a nervous eye on the driver until they were going downhill, following the winding road that brought them to a rocky path leading to the river. They got out of the taxi and Kat pushed crumpled dollars into the driver's hand while Ben fluffed around for his wallet. The air was heavy with heat as she guided him down the rocky path.

'Listen,' Kat said with a wide smile, pulling him by the hand. 'Can you hear that magical sound? Don't you love it? It's my favourite sound in the whole of God's universe.'

'What sound?' asked Ben distractedly. With his free hand he frantically fanned at the mosquitoes and other tiny insects flying towards his face. Kat halted suddenly, looking slightly exasperated.

'What?' Ben shrugged, grinning. He was getting used to the incredulous looks she threw his way so quickly after he replied to her questions.

'The river! Can't you hear the river?'

Ben laughed. 'Oh yeah, the river. What a wonderful sound… that whoosing thing, I mean sound… it's incredible… unbelievable… really amazing.'

Kat shook her head in mock despair and laughed along with him. 'You've got that right, it is incredible.'

The tall bamboo trees that lined the path did little to

keep the glaring sun at bay. Kat explained that the area was eco-protected and little had been done to secure comfort for either natives or tourists. The huts that offered natural fruit, herb juices and vegetarian meals were open plan with no doors or windows, just a roof of sorts.

'As you see there's no electricity so by 5pm the atmosphere is transformed into something dark and eerie. The locals love to spin a *duppy*, or ghost story after dark, but we will be long gone by that time,' she explained, answering his unasked question.

The fresh smell of the river mixed with the scent of earth filled his nostrils. Ben couldn't help smiling to himself. He found it impossible not to compare Kat to Claire-Louise. Kat was so bohemian, while Claire-Louise was such a lady. It fascinated and scared him that he was attracted to two such different women.

Kat stripped down to her underwear, white lace bra and light blue cotton knickers, showing no signs of embarrassment. Claire's underwear would be matching, he thought as he tried to avoid looking at Kat. The level of comfort displayed by Jamaican women of all shapes and sizes towards their bodies still surprised him. He looked around. It seemed that this was a favourite spot for the locals to actually take a bath because there were many people who were washing themselves with soaps and wash cloths, some even shampooing their hair and scrubbing clothes.

'Remember to give something to the river goddess before you get in or she will take something from you. I brought some coral.' She handed him a few pieces. 'Now throw it in or the river goddess will take something from you.'

'I'll risk it.' He laughed at what he considered her superstition and threw the coral into the bushes.

'You standing there all day or what? Come taste the river, it will cool you down.' She splashed water towards him and he jumped back.

'You scared?' she laughed. 'It's been a long time since I've bathed in the river, come join me.'

Ben took off his sandals and jeans, revealing his boxers. He peeled off his shirt and placed it in his rucksack at a safe distance from the river. He walked closer to the river bed, timidly placing a foot forward, withdrawing it with a loud yell.

'Don't be such a child, the water is fresh,' she assured him, holding out a hand.

'I don't think I know anyone who laughs as much as you.' He took hold of her hand and entered the water. It was cold on his hot skin but he felt a gush of warm water periodically. He said just so to Kat who nodded.

'This spot is where the river meets the sea, so the warmth you're feeling is the sea water and the cold is the river.'

Holding hands, joking and laughing, they walked down naturally formed stone steps with gushing waters cooling and massaging their feet. She splashed him, wetting his chest and making him gasp as the cold water hit his skin.

'Right! This means war!' he shouted, holding her hands firmly as he started splashing her with his feet. She laughed even more as their playful water fight erupted.

'I can't remember the last time I laughed so much,' he said as they crawled out of the river.

Kat pulled on her shorts and vest top, shivering so much that Ben wrapped his shirt around her.

'You're cold. There's a soup vendor over there, you want some of your favourite red pea soup to warm you up? I know it's not Ras Solomon's special, but it smells good.'

She nodded and he returned promptly with a steaming cup.

'Ben, look!' she shrieked.

He turned to see a sneaky wave claim one of his sandals.

'You should have given something to the river goddess... now she take it from you.'

Looking down at his feet, then at the stony path they had to walk before reaching the road for a taxi, he grimaced.

'How come it didn't take from you?' he complained.

'I gave her corals, remember. I always bring a gift for the river goddess.'

'Of course you would.' Ben couldn't hide his sarcasm. 'It would make perfect sense to you.'

Once in the taxi, her shivering body seemed to be heating up. Ben automatically pulled her close.

'You feel hot. Maybe you caught a chill staying so long in that river that stole my sandals.'

She wanted to be dropped off in the town and make her own way home but Ben insisted on at least chartering a taxi to take her directly to her door. He wanted to accompany her but thought it best to wait for an invitation. His adoptive father's words echoed in his ear. *Enthusiasm is the gas of life, step on it, but keep your feet on the brake of self-control.* The way he was feeling about her, the warmth that was spreading through him, the need, the urge called for every ounce of self-control he possessed.

'See you same time, same place for another of your adventures.' He pecked her cheek and held her close a moment longer before finally letting her go.

Eight

Miss Ruthie

Miss Ruthie was not happy. In fact she was livid. Not only had Kat returned home in damp clothes, she had the impudence to arrive in a man's shirt and tell her mother to stop fretting. When would her daughter take her condition seriously? Did she forget so soon the hospitals, tubes and needles that she hated so much? Why wouldn't she take her Aunt Doris' experience seriously?

'Kat, what was you doing?' cried Miss Ruthie, following her daughter down the hall.

'I was enjoying life, Miss Ruthie,' explained Kat simply, not in a mood to argue with her mother.

'Then do something that will prolong it, not cut it short.'

Miss Ruthie watched from the entrance of Kat's bedroom, arms folded, a grim look occupying her face as Kat slowly peeled off the damp clothes.

'Let me be, Miss Ruthie, I'm too tired to argue with you.'

'Your ears are too hard, child. When sickness take you who has to nurse you? What you was doing? Why your clothes so wet?'

'I went bathing in the river—'

'You did what!' Miss Ruthie's eyes opened in terror. 'What possessed you? You mad or what? Your father work so hard to get you educated in that school and all you can do is show how fool-fool you is? Sickness will take you for sure!'

'I think you're right, Miss Ruthie. I overdid things this time but I had a whole heap of fun.' She chuckled at the memory as she stiffly snuggled under the covers of her bed.

Miss Ruthie huffed. 'You take bad things to make joke!'

Kat's restlessness and groaning during the course of the night caused Miss Ruthie to send Tim-Tim, her neighbour's son, to fetch Mother Cynthy as morning broke.

'Tell her Kat catch the sickness again,' she told him, handing him fifty dollars. 'And go straight there before you spend the money!'

The young boy ran off bare-footed on thin legs, the fifty dollar bill clasped tightly in his fist.

Miss Ruthie fed the chickens and packed the fruits and vegetables on the table ready for the day's business. She then eased herself into her rocking chair. Samson, the Labrador, joined her, snuggling by her feet. She knew he would lay there until she fed him but he would have to wait until Mother Cynthy came to put her mind at ease about Kat.

'Morning, Miss Rootie.' Nellie's call interrupted Ruthie's thoughts. The woman's sight was never a welcome one, but Ruthie felt even more on edge due to

Kat's illness.

'And to you, Nellie Potato.' She forced herself to be pleasant, even if she knew Nellie had nothing but venom on her tongue.

'A dozen lime and half dozen eggs please,' ordered Nellie Potato, limping through the gate with a plastic bowl.

Miss Ruthie took the bowl and filled it with the requested items.

'I see Old Man Jaguar earlier, you nevah see him pass by here? He was carrying a scandal bag, not sure what was in it though.'

'I have better things doing than to watch people bizness,' Ruthie told her curtly.

'He was carrying the bag like it have something important in. I wonder what him have in it?' She peered at her neighbour suspiciously.

'Anything else?' Ruthie asked, ignoring her insinuation.

'How much for the bunch of Callaloo? Mr Tom might want some for Sunday breakfast.'

'The price don't change since yesterday.'

'Give me two bunch. Old Man Jaguar was talking to Carlos, the Cuban travel agent, people say he booking holiday. What you think?'

Miss Ruthie huffed, feeling increasingly irritated by Nellie's comments. 'Nellie Potato, you know I don't watch people bizness. You want to know what Old Man doing, ask him!'

'I just wondering what he have in that bag. Old Man don't carry bag. He put the bottle of rum in him back pocket, he nevah have need for bag.'

'Five hundred and eighty dollars.' Ruthie held out

her hand.

'Lord! The price of living really gawn up!'

'Same as yesterday price, you pay without complaint.'

'I not complaining, Miss Rootie, I just saying.' Nellie Potato handed her the money. 'Old Man might pass by with him bag in a while. Have a good day.' She gathered her bowl and walked off.

Miss Ruthie was left feeling annoyed, as she did with every visit from Nellie Potato. She thought back about what her neighbour said about Old Man Jaguar and went inside to run a comb through her hair before tying her scarf back on. She also rubbed a little Vaseline on her lips and dabbed a touch of her rose water behind her ears. It annoyed her even more that she did that.

Mother Cynthy's distinct form could be seen miles away, with her trademarks basket of herbs balanced on her head and padded apron that added size to her wide waist. She walked down the dusty lane with the casualness of a Sunday morning stroll, acknowledging everyone along the way and having to stop and listen to their latest ailments, offering them a remedy which they gladly paid for.

She finally arrived at Miss Ruthie's to see her friend sitting in her usual spot on the veranda, chewing grains of rice.

'Morning, Miss Rootie, I hear young Kat take to sickness again.'

Miss Ruthie stood up to greet her friend. 'She was groaning like a donkey in labour all thru' the night. She had fever too, but I keep her cool by rubbing her with some of the bush water you leave and bay rum. She sleeping now. Come through and see her.'

'Good. The fever means she sweating out whatever poison in her system and the sleep will give her back strength,' said Mother Cynthy, following the other woman through the house.

When Kat opened her eyes the brightness of the sunlight caused her to close them instantly.

'She's alright, Miss Rootie, she's alright.' Mother Cynthy patted Miss Ruthie's shoulder upon seeing the alarmed expression on her friend's face.

Kat struggled to sit up but found her head felt as light as whisked egg whites.

'Drink please,' she croaked.

Mother Cynthy disappeared and came back with a discoloured glass of water which she held while Kat took small sips.

'You have a little infection, nothing to cause worry or that needs strong medication but your mother call me in jus' to make sure you alright. You keep to your bed today, gather some strength and in a few days everything fine again.'

She finished the water before Mother Cynthy's words sunk into her. She could not stay in bed for a few days. Ben was waiting for her at the beach.

'I have to go out.' She tried getting up but fell back onto the bed.

'You not going no place. Don't you understand that you been sick? Now is not de time for stubbornness, Kat. You need to rest so your body can heal.'

Tears filled Kat's eyes at her mother's truth-filled words. Her mind may have made the demand but her body wouldn't allow her to just get up and go.

'It's not the same day leaf drop to river bottom it rots. You been going off and staying out till well past evening dew for the last couple days. No wonder you catch infection.'

Defeat swallowed Kat like the waves from the sea.

'Come and drink some mint tea with me on the veranda, Mother Cynthy.'

'Thanks.' Mother Cynthy turned to Kat with a wink. 'Never you mind, Kat. Anything Master God set in stone can't be removed.'

The two women went out and sat on the veranda, sipping their tea in silence before Mother Cynthy interrupted Ruthie's train of thought. 'What riding your mind?'

'Oh, Mother Cynthy,' Miss Ruthie breathed. 'You were so right about Kat being a wild child with a stubborn streak and a strong will. She jus' always follow her unruly mind.' Miss Ruthie could not help feeling protective of her daughter, no matter her age. The worry of a mother never went away.

'Like most pickney,' reasoned the healer. 'She have to find her own way, but she will be alright.'

'What you see, Mother Cynthy? You know something?'

'I know only that Kat will be alright.'

'So you did see something?' insisted Miss Ruthie, grabbing her friend's hand.

'You know I reveal visions only to the person concerned.'

'You dream Kat? What you dream?'

'Behave now, Miss Rootie, behave,' replied the unmovable Mother Cynthy.

Ruthie conceded to defeat. She knew her friend

would not reveal anyone's premonition to a third party. In that sense Mother Cynthy was a true doctor.

'Nellie Potato pass by earlier, talking about Old Man carrying scandal bag. She heated to know what in the bag.'

'A thief never like to see another thief carry a big bag.'

'She don't change over all them years. She still nosey like sin and always wishing bad on people. If she would mind her husband's bizness like she mind everybody else's, he couldn't sleep with every widow or divorcee like he does,' spat Ruthie.

'Don't mind her,' Cynthy advised. 'The Lord wear pyjamas but him don't sleep! She will get her just reward.'

It was mid-afternoon before Old Man Jaguar showed his face, waiting outside the gate under the shade of the almond tree. Miss Ruthie was busy serving customers when he arrived and her hands automatically went to adjust the scarf on her head. He waited until she was free and alone before hesitantly coming into the front yard. Nellie Potato had been right, he had a scandal bag gripped tightly and despite herself her curiosity rose. She busied herself displaying the mangos, oranges and limes that were left.

'Good day, Miss Rootie. How this wonderful day find you?'

'Fine,' she huffed, pretending as she always did with Old Man Jaguar that he was nothing more than annoying.

'I hear Miss Kat take to sickness—'

'She fine now. Mother Cynthy pass by with herb tea and Kat feel better already.'

'I glad to hear that. I not staying long, have to rush to work. I jus' want to leave this.' He held out the scandal bag. 'I hope you don't mind my liberty. An Italian tourist let me choose something for my hard work on the beach and I see it and think 'bout you.'

Ruthie briefly scanned her surroundings before she accepted the bag, just in case Nellie Potato was loitering nearby. She was too proud to open it in front of him and put it to one side as though it was of no importance. Old Man stared at her wordlessly for a few seconds before tipping his hat and walking away.

Once he was safely out of sight, Ruthie took the bag into her house and peered inside it like an excited teenager. It was a pastel pink chiffon scarf with a label that read 'Made in Italy.' The feeling of warmth embraced her like a pair of invisible arms. Pink was her favourite colour and Italy the country she yearned to visit, having only heard about it on the World Service. She always wanted to go and see the Pope and Vatican City, that holiest of places and Old Man knew that. She smiled. It was becoming increasingly difficult to resist him and his impish ways.

Nine
Kat

The following morning Kat stood on the veranda looking towards the rain-threatening sky, host to the dark swollen clouds which she knew would explode any minute. When the first drops came they were bulbous, flattening as soon as they made contact with the ground. The chickens waddled underneath the house and Samson, the Labrador, was beside her under the shelter of the veranda in two leaps. The streets were deserted in the Meadows when it rained. Everyone stayed home, cooking, eating or making love. The rain was always unpredictable because no-one knew how long it would last. Some days it visited for a few minutes, but during the rainy season it could stay for weeks.

Kat sighed audibly as her thoughts wandered to Ben. She could not help the sadness that filled her at the thought of not seeing him another day. She considered phoning Meadow Inn, the guest house he was staying at, but until she collected what was owed to her from her customers she could not buy phone credit. If she used the post office phone, it would give the proprietor, Nellie Potato, gossip to feed the whole town for a year. And Miss Ruthie would not be forgiving of such indiscretion.

Kat sat in the rocking chair, her hands tightly clasped in prayer. If the rain persisted for the day it would mean she could not venture down to the beach and would not see Ben.

'You looking like you have the weight of the world on your shoulders. What you considering so hard?'

She jumped. She had not heard the squeak of the door as Miss Ruthie joined her on the veranda. She quickly came up with a lie to tell her mother.

'I'm just wondering when the rain's going to ease, I need to see Paula before she leaves, I have to get down to the beach,' said Kat, cursing herself for being unable to hide the desperation she felt from her voice.

'You better just forget that beach for today. By the look of the sky Master God has more rain in store.' Miss Ruthie eased herself in her rocking chair, positioning it to face Kat.

'Walking in the rain is therapeutic. I could take an umbrella.'

Miss Ruthie looked at her daughter incredulously. 'You taking leave of your senses? It might well and good be terrorputic for some, but for you it's courting death.' Miss Ruthie rolled the word on her tongue like a weapon. 'You don't need a sickle crisis during wet weather.'

Kat huffed in annoyance. 'Why at any opportunity you want to remind me about crisis and sickness? I'm fully aware of my illness, Miss Ruthie.'

'So you say.'

'How can you say that? I'm the one living with sickle cell! I'm the one feeling the pain, having the drips, the feeding tubes, the...'

'That's where you wrong! Is not just you!' Miss Ruthie interrupted. 'I been living with sickle cell a lot longer than you. There was your daddy before you, plenty, plenty years before you.'

Kat got up. She would usually take heed of her mother's snipes, but Miss Ruthie didn't know the whole story. She wasn't aware of Mother Cynthy's prediction about her becoming a mother or her new relationship with Ben.

'I'll have to miss seeing Paula until she comes back again,' she said instead. She looked up at the sky, feeling drained and discouraged. 'I'm going to lie down.'

'You only just get up. And I hope you don't let that Paula sow any unhealthy seeds in your head. You two always find trouble when your heads knock.'

'We were children then, Miss Ruthie. But she did make me think about travelling, visiting Africa, Namibia where she is.'

'Don't talk trash. Go Africa with your sick self? What doctors they have? Witch doctors? They're not like Mother Cynthy. You forget that thought and now.'

Kat smiled, shaking her head. 'Miss Ruthie, for a Christian you can be very judgemental. My childhood teachings from you was that God made us all. Even Africans.'

Miss Ruthie was right about the rain; it lasted until the following day, finally giving way to the sun. On Friday Kat played lethargic and remained in bed while her mother and their neighbour Mama Gem left for the town to purchase new gas cylinders. As soon as she heard Pa

Gem's old Volkswagen drive off, Kat hopped out of bed and headed outside for her shower. She had to be quick because she knew Miss Ruthie would be fretting about leaving her alone.

She dressed in corn-coloured shorts, rainbow tie-and-dye T-shirt and green flip-flops. She combed her hair back into a pony tail and dabbed a spot of perfume behind her ears. If she hurried she would get to the beach before 2pm and maybe Ben would come. *He must be wondering what happened to me*, she thought. They hadn't exchanged numbers, there was no need, as they had planned to see each other every day until she finished his portrait. Now maybe he went back to Kingston, or worse, back to London believing she no longer wanted to see him. Leaving the house, she grabbed the sketch pad and pencils just in case.

She felt tears rise up as she sat on her stone for two whole hours looking out for the familiar shape, the walk that was all Ben's. The sun had disappeared behind the clouds again and the sky was white and dreary with the breeze periodically whipping up the sand. Her heart felt heavy. The thought that Ben would think badly of her gave her no peace, which caused palpitations to dance like butterflies in her chest. Defeated, she eventually stood up and slowly walked back towards the town centre and her taxi home. Mother Cynthy's prediction had been so close to coming true and now her bubble had been burst. She cried silently, tears escaping down her cheeks. She could not believe she felt such a strong reaction at the thought of never seeing the man from England again. It reinforced her belief that the prediction must have been true—Ben was the man she had been longing for all those years.

She blinked then rubbed her eyes to rid them of the tears and the gritty sand. She continued walking, peering into the distance at a seemingly familiar outline. Suddenly the figure started galloping towards her and waving, and as it got closer she realised it was Ben.

She wished she had the energy to run as he was. She wanted to throw herself into his arms. Then he was there, scooping her up and spinning her around. She dropped her cloth bag with the sketch pad and pencils and clung to him, arms entwined around his neck and her legs lapping his waist.

'Kat... Kat... sweet girl...' He was almost singing her name and she clung to him with all she had. 'Where have you been?' His voice was husky with emotions. 'I came yesterday in the pouring rain, looking for you. I thought you had left me.'

It amazed her that he could ever think that. Fate was once more kind. She should know better than to doubt Mother Cynthy.

'No, never. It wasn't my choice. I've been sick—'

'Sick! I knew it. That day at the river, coming home you were so hot and shivering, you must have caught the flu.'

'Yes, but I'm okay now.'

He placed her gently down. For the first time he could read her eyes. There was no mistaking the words, the feelings, the mood that poured from them.

'Kat...'

'Yes...'

'Sweet girl. Let's go.'

'Yes, quickly, I can smell the rain coming.'

'You can smell rain? Of course you can, what am I thinking even asking that,' he laughed, leading her by the hand.

In the warm and private intimacy of his hotel room, Ben and Kat lay naked in each other's arms. The moment felt surreal to them. It was loud with unspoken feelings. There was no need for words because there were no words to explain their passion. Only the touch of each other's lips, tongues, hands, bodies and breath could fully interpret the moment. And when he lay between her opened thighs, her hips rose to meet his and he took her along with him, rising to touch the stars, to ride the clouds. She gave him her body and he released in her sensations she'd never felt. When his shudder came, she opened her eyes to see such ecstasy all over his face that her pleasure intensified and merged with the unfamiliar tingling storm that consumed her body.

That's what an orgasm feels like, she said to herself.

They lay locked in each other's embrace, both afraid to let go, to untangle limbs in case the moment ended. For the first time in her life Kat believed what people had always said, that she was beautiful despite her sickness.

'Kat...'

'Sshhh. No talk.'

'But I need you to know that... that I'll—'

'Don't forget me.'

'Never. I'll come back; we have to work something out. I have to see you again. Don't you feel what I feel?'

She stroked his face and smiled into him. Her prayers were for the life she hoped they had created.

'Yes.' Her whisper was firm. 'But you live in London

and I live here in the Meadows.'

'So you mean that's it? We don't see each other again after I leave, no phone calls or anything?'

'Who knows what fate has in store for us.' She was thinking, hoping beyond hope that he was the man from the prediction. And their love would make a life.

'I'm not sure I can leave this to fate,' Ben spoke truthfully. 'You've got me, Kat.'

She let out a sigh, pregnant with apprehension. What did that mean? She wanted to ask him. The only thing she knew for sure was the prediction.

'Do I make you uneasy?' Ben questioned.

'No.'

'Then let me have you. What if I buy you a house in Meadow View? I could send you a monthly income, I've—'

Kat looked annoyed and interrupted him. 'Are you serious?'

Ben was flustered. 'Yes.'

'Are you proposing?'

Ben blushed. 'No... of course not. We... we've only just—'

She eased herself onto her elbow and looked down at him.

'Would you ever get married?' She saw the horror that crossed his face and immediately explained herself. 'I don't mean now.' She found his discomfort amusing. 'I was just asking if you'd ever marry in the future.'

He was flustered. 'Yes.' He seemed to dare not say any more. Instead he reached up and smoothed her hair back with one hand.

She was puzzled. Obviously, she thought, he's not

into marriage. If he was he would have married his children's mother. Or maybe she didn't want to marry him, although Kat could not see a reason why any woman on the face of this earth wouldn't want to marry a man like Thornton Benjamin. There was something so unthreatening about him, she couldn't even imagine him having a temper, not with the calmness he emitted.

'Would you ever consider marrying me?' she asked, moving to sit astride him.

She felt his hands on her waist, massaging. 'Yes. Yes. Yes. I would.'

Kat frowned, trying to probe into his mind. 'You sound like you're trying to convince yourself there, with all three yes.'

He didn't respond. Tints of worry flashed in his eyes.

'Anyway, with you living in London, and me in Jamaica, things are going to be difficult. Long distance relationships don't work.'

She knew of such relationships. Holiday romances that courted many promises but which panned out into nothing more than good sex with a foreigner. Or there were the few who had seemed lucky enough to have the man send a ticket for them, only to return home after months, sometimes years suffering from shattered dreams.

'Polly-May Perkins, a girl I went to school with, flew out to London with hopes higher than any plane could fly,' she told him, slightly agitated. 'She came home with stories of living in a little square box.' She made the shape with her hands. 'Which was stacked on top of other little boxes with a clear view of the sky. Why? Because the love of her life was not the rich man he pretended to be when she met him in the Meadows. Then he was driving a hired 4x4 Jeep, with gold dripping from his ears, neck and wrists. He had spent the two-weeks holiday taking her out, eating in Hotel Panama and treating her to manicures, designer clothes and the latest hairstyles. But in London, he was supported by the government and sold drugs. He expected Polly to return to Jamaica, swallow drugs and then go back to London where she would shit out the drugs and earn her living. Only she was caught by customs in London and sentenced to eight years in prison. She served four before being deported and now most of the people in the Meadows don't talk to her. I would never put myself through something like that... I wouldn't fall for someone who would want to treat me like that.'

Ben's finger tips traced the curve of her waist and he laughed as he looked up at her, her curls loose and disturbed.

'You're such a story-teller, you know that? I didn't know your kind of crazy existed.' He laughed, raising himself up to meet her lips with a series of fast kisses. 'Flew out to London with hopes higher than any plane could fly,' he repeated, chuckling and nibbling her neck. 'Just so you know, I have no desire to see you shit out drugs.'

She had so far held no dreams of flying to far-off countries; her dream was simply the fulfilment of Mother Cynthy's premonition.

'What colour are your eyes?' she asked. 'When I first met you I thought they were hazel, now they look like they have pieces of green in them.'

'I think they change according to how I feel,' he

laughed. 'When I first met you I couldn't read your eyes. You're still a bit of a mystery lady to me.'

She frowned. Three years ago she was laid-up in hospital, going through another sickle attack. Tubes. Transfusions. Pain. And as she lay on the bed all she longed for was the feel of the sand again, so she knew she was still alive. There was no mystery in that.

'You're unreadable again. What are you thinking?' His hand began stroking her body. 'Don't lock me out... let me in.'

'You are in.' Her voice was suggestive as her body responded to his touch.

He flipped her over so that he was now on top. 'I have this insane feeling that we met for a reason,' he whispered in her ear. 'So we just have to figure out what that reason is.' Then his lips came down on hers, sipping and savouring her as though she were a delicious beverage.

Mother Cynthy's premonition flashed in her head, like a car's headlamp alerting an oncoming vehicle. As his kisses became hungrier with passion, there in her core was the greatest feeling of serendipity.

Ten

Ben

The following morning, a telephone call stirred them from their dreams, the insistent ringing like the buzzing of an annoying bee. Ben reached for his mobile phone, knocking it off the bedside table, then fumbled to find it on the floor. Eyes still closed, he finally located it and placed it to his ear. He responded, fighting his way to consciousness. He could tell that the voice he heard was familiar even through the cloud of sleep. A streak of sun streamed across the still dark skies and the crowing of the roosters suddenly jerked him fully awake. The sounds of Jamaica still took some getting used to.

'Ummmm. Hello, hello?'

'Benny boy! Where are you?' said a deep voice on the line.

'Bubs?'

'That's my name. I thought you were going to pick me up from Montego Bay airport, remember I'm staying for the weekend before I fly home.'

'Yes, on the 5th.'

'Then what date do you think it is today?'

Ben jumped up. 'Shit, Bubs, I'm on my way.'

He hung up, then turned to Kat, who was awakening from her sleep, a smile seductively perched on her lips.

'Sorry to disturb you, sweet girl, I completely forgot that I have to pick my friend up from the airport. He's there already so I got to rush.' He pulled his shorts on, grabbed a T-shirt and quickly pecked her forehead. 'How can you smell rain coming?' He had wanted to ask her last night.

'The air gets cooler, fresher and the smells of the trees and plants are more potent. The animals tell you also. I better get going too; I have a private sitting so I'll see you later.' Kat yawned, her arms stretched above her head.

Ben stopped at the entrance of the door, shaking his head and smiling back at her. 'Where do you even get these notions from? Smelling rain?'

The drive on the newly-paved road was smooth and swift in the beach buggy Ben hired from the guest house. He had to pay out a little more on top to get the deal at that time of morning, but he was accustomed to the giving of tips to get things going in Jamaica. Anything could be accomplished as long as you had the finance.

The coastal route to the airport was no less than picturesque. Already there were traders along the road selling souvenirs, offering cooked breakfast from fires in tin drums and opened-door wooden shacks stacked high with fruits and juices too irresistible to pass by. Ben stopped, thinking Bubs had waited this long so he could wait a bit longer. He purchased a jelly coconut and three mangos and was somewhat surprised to see the vendor was Dollar-Galore.

'Mr Ben!' The lanky teenager looked genuinely pleased to see him.

'Hey, Galore, or should I call you Percy?'

'Drop the Percy... you and me is bredren so Galore is all good!'

Ben drank the jelly down thirstily. 'This is your shop?' he asked in between sips.

'No, sah. It belong to mi uncle but him sick today and sometimes I help him out.'

Galore put forward his foot. 'See my new trainers, I buy them with the money you gave me. They look good, don't?'

Ben nodded and laughed. 'Well, I'd better be on my way.'

Galore had that look on his face again, the one Ben saw the first time he met him. The one that warned he was going to offer a deal. 'You on your way to the port to pick up?'

'Yes, my best friend from school days,' Ben announced proudly.

'You passing back this way, sir?'

'Oh yes. He'll be staying in the Meadows with me.'

'Don't you find the Meadows quiet? Not much action unless you're into church. If you want action I can show you one nice little shack called Off the Beaten Track. It offer everything a foreigner could want.' He lowered his tone to a whisper. 'Ganja or something stronger, pretty girls, over proof rum... anything you want I can get.'

'Thanks,' Ben laughed. 'I'm sure my friend would appreciate that... if time permits.'

Bubs was all muscle and smiles as he bounced out of the

arrivals with the bop of a rapper, an attendant pushing his suitcase on a trolley. His smile widened as he caught sight of Ben and he saluted. He was stocky with cheeky twinkling brown eyes and a wide grin, which was a constant even when he was speaking. His wild brown hair stood straight, as though he had received an electric shock and his aura was infectious and inviting.

'Hey, Benny, my boy—look at you! That sun has sure been kissing your arse, given you a bit of black on that brown skin of yours.'

'Hey, Bubs!' Ben embraced his friend. 'I've kind of missed your big mouth! Follow me, I'm parked over there,' he pointed.

The attendant lifted the case with ease into the boot and waited dutifully until Ben gave him his monetary tip.

'Let's hit the road, Benny boy, I want to change out of these clothes then hit the famous rum bars... and of course any pretty girls you can line up.'

'What about letting me know how the job went, and how did you land it? Landscaping for the rich, that's the dream.'

'Ain't no mystery in that, Benny boy. My mother's friend from Miami was staying for a few days and she fell in love with the garden. She also just happens to work for the Oprah Winfrey Network and of course Mum boasted about her landscape gardener son who designed it, and the old girl paid me to do hers in Miami.'

Traffic had built up and it was a bumper to bumper drive all the way back to the Meadows. Ben did not dare stop off to see Galore for fear of having to re-enter the jam. It took two and a half hours before he was back in the Meadows.

After booking into his own Bubs relaxed in his best friend's room at the guest house. Showered and dressed in the elaborate uniform of tourists—patterned shorts and white string vest—he sipped his Jack Daniel's with sheer satisfaction.

'You know, despite the co-ordinating colours with these matching cushions and curtains, the rooms lack a woman's touch. It's too formal,' Bubs criticised.

Ben toyed with the glass of rum punch ordered from room service in his hand, thoughtfully looking at the huge picture of the beach that took centre stage on the wall.

'Guest houses are temporary accommodation, Bubs, they're not designed to feel like home,' he responded absentmindedly.

'I got something for you, wait a mo'!' Bubs rushed out of the room and was back in seconds.

'Hey, Benny, how'd you like this?' He held up a large colourful canvas painting of beautiful women in bikinis on a sun drenched beach. He placed the painting on Ben's lap.

'Next time, you must come to Miami. Everywhere you look you see sun and women, sun and women and wow are they built!' He outlined the shape of a woman with both hands.

Ben looked at the painting and thanked Bubs. 'What about the buildings? The architecture must be quite stunning, a mixture of old and new?'

'Who's got time to look at buildings? The only building that caused me any wonder was how them women's backsides are built! That thought puts everything else out of your fucking mind! Have you ever reeeeally studied them butts?'

Ben laughed.

'And I know you've heard this tons of times before, but I'm in lust-love, Benny Boy, with Sharisa. She's got smooth dark skin, skin dark as Bourneville chocolate and teeth as white as the clouds. She has two huge breasts like melons and a belly as taut as stretched elastic. Not to mention her chunky thighs like a Yorkie chocolate bar. She's delicious like food I'm telling you.'

Ben understood perfectly.

'What about you Benny? Any of them hot Jamaican girls juice you?'

It was delivered as a joke and Ben tried to hide his reaction but Bubs had known him for too many years not to have been alerted by the sight of Ben shifting uncomfortably in his chair.

'Holding out on me, bro?' Bubs teased.

Ben felt bashful. He also didn't want to betray Kat by revealing their relationship. And he did think of Kat in terms of a relationship, not an affair.

Bubs circled Ben's chair, becoming more intrigued with each second the silence stretched. Ben again shifted uncomfortably in his chair, acutely aware of Bubs scrutiny.

'Come on, bro!' Bubs voice had become impatient. Ben had something to tell and he wanted to hear it. 'Explain! I can hardly wait!'

Placing his drink on the coffee table, Ben slowly rubbed his hands together. It was difficult to talk about Kat. How could he explain what they shared in such a short time? It was important that Bubs understood what he was about to tell him. His friend, Ben had always known, was a player from his mother's womb. He had never been serious about any of the long list of girls he had dated and bedded over the years. He had broken more hearts than Casanova, Don Juan or any other historical or present day super lover. Love just wasn't logical to Bubs. Ben sighed. Impatience now rampant, Bubs pulled a stool and sat facing Ben, his eyes tunnelling with frenzy into his friend's.

'I saw her long before she saw me. At first I wasn't sure why I kept watching her sitting crossed-legged on the beach,' he laughed at the memory. 'I think it was her stillness. The fact that she was still for so long had me wondering if she was real, you know.'

Bubs shook his head. 'No, I don't know.' He drew the stool closer, his eyes now bright with fascination.

Ben continued, 'She sat in the same place at the same time every afternoon and I sat watching her for a few days before I actually talked to her.' He took a sip of his drink and placed it down again.

'Days? Fucking days to talk to a woman! Now why doesn't that surprise me about you?' Bubs shook his head in mock dismay.

'She turned out to be more real than I expected.'

'Shit! Benny, what are you saying?' Bubs was opened-mouthed and incredulous. 'You're the only man I know who can be called faithful, bro.'

They had known each other from the age of ten and in the twenty-four years of their friendship Bubs had proved to be fun, the player and Ben sober, the devoted. No amount of Bubs pleading or teasing could make Ben join him and the other guys in group sex with a few party-loving girls.

'Her name's Katherine St Monica Lewis, or Kat. She's...' he trailed.

'What?' Bubs prodded.

'She's an artist. A real beauty and has this spark, passion, this intellect that excite me.' He stood up and started pacing the room. 'She's deep, Bubs, she thinks about things like other universes and believes in river goddesses and can even smell rain coming—she takes me out of this world.'

Bubs suddenly jumped up throwing his arms in the air in disgust.

'Oh shit, Benny boy! Don't give me the fucking choir boy point of view, was she hot? How the fuck did she get a fuddy-duddy like you to free it up? What was she like in bed, man?'

'You know I don't kiss and tell,' smirked Ben.

'Fuck you! No wonder you forgot what date it was... good pussy does that.'

They both laughed, Bubs viewing his friend through interest-soaked eyes. Ben knew he had astonished Bubs. He had even astonished himself with this riot of passion and emotions that meandered through his veins at the thought of her, still very much a stranger to him, yet a mate of his soul he felt he'd known for an eternity. It would be impossible to explain this. Bubs would probably never, in this lifetime or the next, understand such a concept and neither would he want to.

'Well, I don't feel so bad about me now,' Bubs announced. 'If you can fall off the wagon, ain't no man in the whole of this universe fucking loyal.'

'I'm always reminding you I'm no angel,' Ben pointed out, taking another sip of his drink.

'Yeah, but I never fucking believed you. I mean you settled with the first woman you had good sex with and wanted nothing to do with any other woman. I personally don't know another man like you... only you're kinda like me now... you're naaaasty!' Bubs couldn't help having a dig and Ben expecting it received it in good humour.

The past week spent with Kat had seemed like he was journeying without a destination. There was no-one to tell about her, to seek advice from and help him analyse his new feelings, feelings that were so alien and so exhilarating. Bubs had been in London and the phone an unsuitable option to spill his woes, too impersonal and off-putting when he couldn't read body language or eyes. Now he had started talking about her, the relief came in floods.

'I know all I have is a week left. I haven't allowed my mind to consider beyond that time, but I'll have to. I'm falling deeper and deeper into her and it's out of my control.'

'A whole lot of bed work can take place in a week,' Bubs sniggered.

'It's not just about sex, Bubs.' Ben sounded annoyed.

'Seriously now, what is it about? Why her?'

Ben shrugged. 'There's something about her... something. She's a bit of a bohemian but I'm a different man with her, not better, just different, Bubs, and I like that difference. I just like it.'

'Bohemian, nice, they can be real freaky... Is she good looking?'

'She's beyond good looks.'

'What the fuck does that mean? Ugly?'

'No. It means she's beautiful; because being kind,

warm-hearted, funny, intelligent, all these qualities equal beautiful and sexy to me.'

'I can honestly say with my hands on my heart that I've never fucking felt like that about any woman, not even my baby mothers... don't suppose I ever will.'

Bubs gulped down the remainder of his drink. 'One word, Benny boy: Claire.'

Claire-Louise and the children. Ben had so far managed to keep from facing reality and really wasn't ready to start now.

'I haven't told Kat about Claire. She knows about the children... She's satisfied with so little and extremely independent... I wanted to help her, buy her a decent home but she won't even consider that.'

'And good for her! You can't go round feeling obligated to every woman who gives you a good fuck—it's suicide. And how you going to explain buying a house in Jamaica to your wife?'

Ben didn't look convinced.

'It's not a good idea to get stuck on a fling, Benny.'

'She's not a fling, Bubs.'

'It would be for the best if you viewed her as a fling. You've had her, now forget her.'

Ben sighed in gloom. He knew Bubs wouldn't understand. He hadn't expected him to, but it was just so liberating to be able to talk about his feelings for her to someone. It gave him a chance to work out for himself what had happened to him and what he was going to do about it.

'Look, bro,' Bubs continued, 'when you start playing "outdoors" you gotta think smart. You can't afford to be stuck on any one woman if you still want your marriage to work or your wife will feel it. Women have some extra senses that tells them things about us, don't you know! They're kind of like witches.'

He knew alright. Claire's phonecalls had become more regular since he met Kat. She had the uncanny knack of phoning when Kat was entertaining his thoughts.

'I'll do you a big favour. Now you've ventured outside Claire's bed, I'll have a discreet word in Mandy's ears. Hey, every time I see that chick she asks if you're still with stuck-up Claire whose shit don't stink. She confessed that you set her skin on fire and when I was trying to get me a piece of her, she had the fucking nerve to tell me you're the only man in West London she'd fuck. Man that really hurt because I know you'd refuse it!'

'I didn't set out to–to bed or... even love her.' Not consciously. He didn't know how it had all happened and he didn't want to know. He knew only that he wanted her and would try his best to keep her.

'Fuck's sake! Who's talking about love? Listen, friend.' Bubs placed two firm hands on Ben's shoulders. 'You're new to this cheating shit, so let me give you a bit of advice. You don't need to feel guilty. A man can love his fish, chips and mushy peas, but it doesn't mean he wants it every day. He might want a little rice and peas and brown stew chicken—you get me. Enjoy it while it lasts because after next week you're back to the true you, a husband with a wife and two kids.'

Eleven

Kat

Kat was in a hurry when she met with Ben in Meadows Inn's reception that afternoon. Tucked under her arm was a large rectangular package, which she explained she had to drop off at the Craft Market for a customer. Her hair, which in all truth could have done with some tidying up, was in a ponytail and she donned yellow denim shorts with a plain white T-shirt, and her trademark flip-flops on her feet.

'I have a family portrait to finish, so I'll be working into the evening.' She smiled apologetically. 'I'll still come, so wait up.'

He held on to her hand. 'I want you to meet someone, it will only take a minute,' he promised, leading her through to the dining area, where the aroma of some jerked meat filled her nose, causing her tongue to involuntarily run across her lips.

He walked her over to a table where a muscular man sat, sinking his teeth into a chicken leg.

'Kat, this is Bubs, my best and most annoying friend. Bubs, this is Kat.'

Bubs placed the half-eaten chicken leg on the plate

and swiftly wiped his hand on the white table cloth, leaving the brown residue of the jerk.

'Hi, pleased to meet you,' Kat smiled somewhat surprised as she looked at Ben.

'Nice meeting you, Kat... won't shake hands, you understand?' He held both hands up, the remnants of the jerk sauce still evident. 'Are you going to join us for lunch? Only I want to get to know you, the girl that's stolen my friend's heart.' His smile was wide, revealing impressive white teeth, the front two slightly over lapping and adding an unusual charm to his chubby face.

Kat shook her head, Bubs' eyes seemed to hold hers a second longer than was comfortable. 'Afraid not, I have a portrait I have to finish but I'll take you guys to the Falls tomorrow if you like.'

'I love,' Bubs said, and before she turned to go she thought again that his eyes were trying to see something beyond her face.

She hesitated, not sure what to make of him—the cheeky eyes that flirted with laughter and mischief. Was it her he was laughing at? She couldn't be certain but at least he didn't make her uncomfortable and she found herself drawn to him. His accent, although English was harder to understand than any English person's she had ever met. Ben had explained that Bubs spoke a mixture of cockney and Jamaican Patois, which she disputed. His Patois could not be called Jamaican. He was shorter than Ben, but bigger in body size and wore sandals without socks. She could tell that Bubs enjoyed letting the devil loose in his mind. Her mother's adage, 'Show me your friends and I'll tell you who you are' would be incorrect against Ben's rather reserved manner. She wondered how they had become friends in the first place.

She began the morning as she usually did by setting out the fruits and vegetables on the table in front of their house, and collecting the eggs from the chickens, which would bring in their daily income. She then fed the chickens and Samson before taking her morning shower. She sang at the top of her voice, happiness had never felt so sweet. She allowed the water from the hose pipe to trickle down her body, caressing places Ben had touched so tenderly the night before. She had never felt as alive as the moments she spent with him. She slipped her wet feet into her rubber slippers and grabbed a towel, wrapping it snugly around her body; it felt like Ben's comforting hugs. She emerged from the bathroom to come face to face with her mother, a scowl scarring her face.

'Morning, Miss Ruthie.' She slid past, ignoring the tell-tale sign of disapproval and ran up the back stairs into the house and her room. She patted herself dry and reached for the coco butter, smoothing it over her skin in slow, sensuous strokes, emulating Ben's hand movements. There were no doors to any of the rooms in the house; just curtains which served as partitions and were supposed to offer privacy.

'You been looking mighty pleased with yourself these past few weeks. He sweet you so?' Miss Ruthie had swept the curtain to one side and was standing obstructively, arms folded across her bosom, the scowl a mark of annoyance.

'Miss Ruthie, why don't you let me know when you're entering my space?' Kat grabbed the towel to hide her nakedness.

'What? When since I have to?' she queried, obviously offended. 'And what you hiding? I been seeing you naked since birth, you never had a problem with it before, but suddenly you hiding like you think I'm some stranger.'

Kat grasped for an answer that simply would not emerge. She was usually one step ahead of her mother's banter, enquiries or criticisms, but they had never come at a time when her body had been devoured and completely obsessed by love, passion and the deepest desire. She felt intimate and treasured. She wanted to share her nakedness with no-one but Ben. She was absolutely sure no woman had been so loved.

For once she was totally lost for words and felt her mind as well as her body could be read by Miss Ruthie. She felt her mother could see the hands that had caressed her, making her moist and sensuous, and read her mind, hearing the words whispered in her ears at the height of heated passion.

'Can I just dress in private, please, Miss Ruthie?'

Miss Ruthie turned and marched out of the small room and Kat picked out her jeans and blue lace cotton blouse. She looked at her small selection of clothes, ironed and folded neatly in the chest of drawers. She had never before wanted or wished for clothes. There had always been far more important things to think about other than new garments to parade in. Now she wished she had more sophisticated clothes to wear on her days out with Ben. She laughed at herself in the mirror and mouthed, *You're a winner!*

She inhaled deeply before leaving her room. There was no doubt Miss Ruthie would be in a disagreeable mood. She took small steps into the living room where Miss Ruthie stood with a white shirt dangling from one finger. It was Ben's. The shirt she had worn home the evening of her illness.

'Does this by any chance have anything to do with your secretive behaviour?'

Kat grabbed the shirt with annoyance. 'Why are you searching my belongings?' she accused.

'What?' Miss Ruthie barked. 'Let me tell you something, I never search nothing! You put this in the wash basket and I washed it!'

Kat began folding the shirt because there was nothing else she could do to ease the awkwardness she felt.

'You want to tell me what happening? Why you get so secretive?'

No, she didn't.

'You have a boyfriend?'

'Boyfriend? No. I'm twenty-eight, Miss Ruthie, I wouldn't date a boy.'

'So you have a man?'

Kat's silence did nothing to halt the questions.

'Who is it? Not Columbus? Not Curtis, Miss Bertie's bwoy? Them two run behind you like bee round honey pot, but I don't see you pay them no serious mind.'

'It's none of them, Miss Ruthie. You know Columbus has gone back to Paris and Curtis is dating Marlene Harris and if you remember, his mother told him not to date a sickling like me.' She wanted to add that Curtis had persuaded her to give up her virginity then promptly told her that he couldn't get serious with her because his mother wanted grandchildren, and everyone knew Kat Lewis was not going to be able to bear children.

'Then is who?'

'His name is Ben, he's from London.'

'A foreigner!' Miss Ruthie screeched. 'You take leave of your senses or what? Those men only use Jamaican girls, he'll have you swallow drugs which burst in your belly and kill you or get you lock up in foreign jail or worse still, breed you!'

'He's not into drugs, Miss Ruthie. He's sort of an architect... well more of a realtor.' Kat hesitated. 'He has an eye for designs and oversees building projects and he sells them after they're completed.' She paused for a beat. 'I'll invite him round.'

'No you won't! I not having no foreigner come and criticise my humble home, look down on us, you a poor country girl.'

'Ben is not like that, Miss Ruthie. You need to meet him. Maybe you come out with us. Make no more judgements until you meet him. You'll love him, I promise you.'

Miss Ruth pointed an accusing finger. 'If you doing any funny bizness with him, you go and see Dr Mattie or Mother Cynthy. You can't have no babies, Katherine St Monica Lewis, you hearing me!'

'You don't always know God's plan,' she snapped. 'Just let me be happy if only this once, and meet him,' she called calmness back into her voice. 'He's so sweet, Miss Ruthie.'

'Mind what sweet you don't sour you!' Miss Ruthie warned solemnly.

Mother Cynthy was at the end of her rounds when Kat saw her heading towards the road leading up into the hills. The strangest thing about Mother Cynthy was that you always saw her when you needed her the most and she was never surprised at seeing you. It was as if she expected you. It was nearing afternoon and Kat had left Miss Ruthie to carry out the selling of their provisions, surrounded by the usual flurry of customers, with Old Man hanging outside the gate and Nellie Potato eyeing him suspiciously. Kat hurried, calling after the old lady. Mother Cynthy heaved the full basket off her head with ease, resting it by her feet and waited for Kat.

'Good day, Kat, what's your gripe?'

'Good day, Mother Cynthy. Miss Ruthie,' Kat replied, dejectedly.

Mother Cynthy laughed, the raucous sound coming from her jerking belly.

'It's no joke—she keeps reigns on me like an unruly donkey.'

This caused Mother Cynthy to laugh even more. She beckoned for Kat to follow her as she perched on the low stone wall that separated the dirt road from the bush leading to the hills. Kat sat beside her, eager to remove the weight of complaint from her chest. The old lady wiped her brow with the piece of cloth she pulled from one of the pockets on her apron.

'Your mother has been doing that ever since… so what's your real gripe?'

'I've met him, Mother Cynthy. The man from across the sea who will make a baby with me. I–I think I like him a lot, and I told Miss Ruthie about him and she's getting ready to flap like a headless chicken.'

'Souls that are meant to be must cross paths. Miss Rootie can't stop that,' Mother Cynthy spoke looking intently at Kat. 'Is your blood late?'

'It isn't due yet. I invited Miss Ruthie to meet him but because he's a foreigner, she refused. All she sees is a drug don who'll put me to work.'

'I didn't see that, but I sense a man with secrets, as I told you.'

'We all have secrets, Mother Cynthy. I haven't told him about my sickle because I don't want him to treat me differently. I don't want anyone to know about us right now.'

'You can hide and buy land but you can't hide and work it!'

'First I've heard that one?' Kat said with a smile.

'You can hide and have a relationship but you can't hide the baby produced from it—the truth will be revealed.'

Kat reached for an orange from Mother Cynthy's basket. Her mouth felt dry and the juice from the fruit gave relief. 'I think he likes me as much as I like him. I just want to be sure he's not a user. I want to be sure about him, Mother Cynthy. What else do you see for me?'

'Oh there is always much more than I see. Much more.'

Twelve

Kat

The week had grown wings. In another three days Ben would be flying home to London. It was also his friend Bubs' last night of holiday and Kat had promised to take them to the Falls, but it began to rain. The rain in the Meadows could be amazing. Sometimes the skies wouldn't darken, but remain clear blue and cloudless, yet the raindrops could be the size of fists, turning roads into streams in minutes. And then just as suddenly as it started, it would stop and the sun would burn hot and evaporate the pools of water. But this time the lightening split the skies and the rain poured down relentlessly like when Noah built the Ark, preventing any movement.

Kat sat in the foyer of Meadows Inn, watching the two friends as they joked and laughed about events she had never been privy to. Their boyish banter gave her the opportunity to see Ben as she had never done before and it pleased her that there was a silly side to him. It fascinated her how he would close his eyes whenever he laughed, or how when the sun shone on him the flecks of green in his eyes became prominent. There were so many physical characteristics she loved about him.

'You should have known this guy at twelve, Kat. You would never believe how troublesome he was. He actually tried to burn our school down.'

She looked at Ben in astonishment. 'Ben, burn down a building? But he loves buildings!'

'Not when he was twelve. He was criminal. He lived to torture... but mostly himself. He was an angry little shit.'

Bubs, she thought, had the ability to chuckle like a mischievous monkey.

'No need to take him too seriously,' Ben offered apologetically, 'he can't help himself.'

'We have a saying here in Jamaica: see me and come live with me and you'll find two different people.' She peered at Ben, savouring his smile and falling deeper.

'Oh you'll be surprised at what you'll find if you come and live with this one.'

Bubs slapped Ben's shoulder.

Kat was swift to see the annoyed glare Ben threw at Bubs, who simply howled with wide-mouthed laughter. It was the first time since meeting Ben that she actually thought deeper about Mother Cynthy's words; *he holds secrets.*

'Ever thought of visiting London, Kat? Has Ben invited you?'

'No, I've never thought of visiting London. Any place cold doesn't appeal to me.' Her answer was measured as she wondered what undertone lay in his voice.

'Oh, really?' Bubs looked unconvinced. 'Most Jamaican girls would sell body and soul for that opportunity. To get a visa and go to London is a dream come true.'

'Most are not me.' She looked at Ben, searching for

reactions and found the look of a school boy caught in his guilt.

'Can I be blatant?' Bubs, now merry with rum punch and Red Stripe beer, questioned.

'Bubs! What—'

'Let him.' Kat stopped Ben's interruption with a touch on his arm, curious as to where this whole conversation was leading to. 'Blatant is good.'

Bubs nudged Ben playfully. 'Girl has guts, unlike her man.' He chuckled and took a deep breath trying to still the humour he felt at Ben's obvious discomfort. 'I just want to know where your relationship is heading. You don't want to go to London, where incidentally your man lives and works—so what's happening after this? Or is it just a holiday romance? I mean you guys seem all wrapped up in each other, I'm just wondering what the real story is. What next?'

It was the undertones she heard in his voice. It halted her. She turned to Ben questioningly and noticed the flicker of panic in his eyes. The truth was that no plans had materialised in her mind as to what would happen after he left. She was trying so hard not to love him, in case he turned out to be like Polly May's boyfriend, but she couldn't control the way he made her feel when he looked at her. Whenever he touched her or laughed—his eyes questioning and delving, intrusive. She always felt the need to build a shield so that his nosey eyes wouldn't read her. Had Bubs asked this question two weeks earlier her answer would have been instant and different. But now love's roots had curled itself in and around her like a boisterous growth of ivy and she was out of her depth in love. Bubs had opened up a door which would require a shift of mind, a move filled with too much realism.

The warmth of Ben's hand soaked through her thin cotton blouse reassuringly.

'Tell him what's next, Ben.' She laid the responsibility at his feet so she could see where her future lay.

'Next?' Ben repeated. 'Next is that we get out of here and enjoy some of that sun that's just peeped through the clouds.'

She was glad for that response, as she anticipated that Bubs might start asking more pointed questions about her and the secret she did not want to reveal.

Bubs drained his glass and placed it with a bang on the table. 'Like my friend Ben says, Kat, ignore me. I like playing devil's advocate. I'm quite harmless, really. No hard feelings?' His smile was friendly as he held out a hand.

Kat returned the smile, accepting his gesture. 'I don't like hard feelings.'

Bubs left them to walk the beach together. Kat fell into thoughtful silence, a heavy shadow absorbing her like ink on blotting paper, spreading to all the crevices of her mind until she felt she would burst if she didn't voice her concerns. Bubs had opened the floodgate and now questions were begging for answers. She briefly glanced at him, taking in his profile and admiring the chiselled look of his cheek. She knew every detail, every inch of his face which she so enjoyed discovering as he slept after their love making. It was in those secret moments that she assembled the features of the child they would have and visualised the gene his father would pass onto him.

'A penny for them.' Ben interrupted her flow of thoughts.

'Huh?'

'Your thoughts. You're very quiet, want to share?'

She came to a halt and looked up at him. 'I want to ask you something, and I want the truth,' she warned with the sternness of a school teacher. She felt his hand stiffen.

'Fire away.'

'What's your secret? Will it hurt me?'

The look that misted his eyes signalled her defences. She felt she would require a steel armour to deal with whatever he was going to admit. He rested his hands on her shoulders, gently at first and then it turned into a firm massage.

'There's no easy way to say this, so I'm just going to...' he sighed so deep that fear clutched her. He pulled her into his arms. 'Don't hate me and don't leave me.'

She pulled away. 'Why would I?'

After a long intense moment of looking at her, Ben finally admitted, 'I'm married.'

A frown crossed her face. 'Married as in, married-miserable-separated?'

Ben shook his head. 'No. Married, as in married.'

Her silence grew thorns that pricked at his conscience.

She had never felt such confusion. It washed over her like the cold torrent from the river, snatching her breath for a moment so that she had to gasp to get it back. He pulled her into him again and she felt her knees shake, her stomach cartwheel. Her heart break. He was rocking her and talking and she was still fighting to understand his words.

'Sweet girl, forgive me, Kat. I should have told you and I had all intentions to, but I knew once I did you might not want to see me again and the more I saw of you the more I wanted to keep you. I'm hooked. Don't leave me.'

There was a hint of trance in her voice. 'I should know better. Mother Cynthy said you had secrets. You were so uncomfortable when I asked your opinion on marriage. I should have known. Married? You have a wife...' Her voice became a whisper, 'You have a wife, Ben? How could you lie to me about that?'

She pulled herself out of his arms, backing away slowly, her eyes deep with accusation. Then she turned away, as if looking at him was pain itself.

'Don't, Kat. Let's talk about this.' He held on to her shoulders firmly, forcing her to look at him.

She struggled free from his grasp. 'Talk? No. You've lost that privilege. Let me go, I never want to see you again. Bubs, he was trying to read me, find out what kind of woman sleeps with a married man. He must think me so low.'

He followed her as she marched angrily along; she wished he would just disappear before the tears erupted and tempt her to fall against him and drink in his apology like thirst would water, but he was insisting on explaining the unexplainable.

'No, Bubs doesn't think that way about you. We can't end it here; just give me a few minutes, please, Kat.' He attempted to grab her hand.

'Let go of me, don't touch me, go back to your wife! You liar!' she spat.

Mother Cynthy got it all wrong. This was not the

man to father her child, to love her. Her dream dissolved like sugar in water and with it came the tears, the sobs, uncontrollable sobs. Her heart shattered into more tiny grains than the sand beneath her feet and she started to run towards the taxi bay, Ben in close pursuit, pleading his cause.

'Kat? What in heaven's name is this? Why you wailing like a child orphaned?'

Nellie Potato, who was walking by the beach, grabbed at her arm and forced her to a standstill. She looked at Ben with curious eyes before turning back to Kat. 'You want to share a taxi to the Meadows with me? You can tell me all about this.'

Kat brushed Nellie's hand away. 'Let me go, Nellie Potato, just let me be.'

'Kat,' Ben pleaded, 'sweet girl, please, please, let's talk.'

She couldn't bear to be near him. Her mind was suddenly filled with the outline of a woman, the other woman, his wife. Ben had a wife. The stench of betrayal was too suffocating.

'Stay away from me,' she shouted at him, over Nellie Potato's eyes, both wide with curiosity.

Thirteen
Miss Ruthie

'If man don't dead don't call him *duppy*,' Ruthie Lewis barked at Nellie Potato who had arrived for her daily fruits and vegetables extra early.

'But Selma Newton see it with her own eyes. Mr Gilbert on him dead bed and all round him people are going in and helping themselves to him belongings. If him not near dead, him would know. The grim reaper is surely near to take him soul up to heaven...' she lowered her voice, '... or some even say hell!'

Miss Ruthie busied herself packing Nellie Potato's order, unwilling to add to poisonous gossip.

'Anything else I can get you?' She handed her customer the basin of provisions she had ordered.

'No, this is fine. You know people say Mr Gilbert is one hundred and seven years old, he outlive all his relatives, sons, daughters and grandchildren, no-one left to bury him. I hear the village council have to pay for him funeral... what a sad situation. I put money aside for my funeral. I don't want no pauper send-off. When I go to meet the Lord, I want to arrive in splendour. Poor Mr Gilbert—no chick nor child to mourn him.'

Ruthie held on to the urge to question Nellie Potato as to who she thought would mourn her. Certainly not her husband. Farmer Tom had always been more interested in giving comfort to other women. And none of her children, who had all left the Meadows, some living in foreign countries and not sending as much as a Christmas card for her. And none of her grandchildren either, who just used her as a bank, always taking out loans and never repaying her, if she was to be believed.

Ruthie picked up the broom. 'Anything else I can get for you, Nellie Potato?'

'No, thanks, I have to get back to the post office, I leave Miss Jeanie's grand-daughter to mind it for me. Between me and you, she have the common sense of a jackass. I'll be seeing you, Miss Rootie.'

Nellie limped to the gate where with a glint in her eye she hesitated before turning around. 'I see young Kat has a beau, a foreigner, walking up and down the beach holding hands'. She squinted over at Miss Ruthie to see if her words had gained any traction. Miss Ruthie's head remained firmly downward adjusting her already orderly produce. Nellie Potato wanted blood. 'Last night he do something to make her cry...' No response. She carried on, slightly miffed, 'I see them with me own eyes on the beach, she was crying like she was a dead woman's child.' There was wedge of silence between them since Miss Ruthie now behaved as if the woman at her gate was invisible. Nellie grabbed at the gate barely containing her frustration. 'Good day to you, Miss Rootie.'

Ruthie felt like Nellie Potato had just punched her in the gut and kicked her in the chest. If Nellie

Potato knew that about Kat, it meant the whole of the Meadows knew too. She climbed the stairs to the veranda as if her slippers were made of iron. Easing herself into the rocking chair she reached for her bag of rice, reflecting on the past few weeks. Kat took greater care of her appearance, everything she wore matched, and she always smelled of the sweet perfume Columbus had brought her back from Paris. Then there was the shirt, the one she wore home the evening sickness took her. A foreign and expensive shirt, with a label that read 'Armani.' These foreign relationships were usually over in a couple of days, weeks and that's why she hadn't wanted to meet him when Kat suggested it. In retrospect she thought perhaps she should have agreed. She may have been able to save Kat the heartache that would eventually engulf her.

'Miss Rootie, your mind fly from you?'

She was lost so deep in thoughts that she had not noticed Old Man Jaguar until he was on the top step of the veranda. He pulled up the stool beside her, removed his hat and placed it on the table.

'You hear about Kat too?' she asked.

He didn't try to conceal anything. 'Yeah man! Miss Kat is all loved up. She look healthy and happy, I glad like Solomon in Sheba's arms for her.'

Miss Ruthie glared at him, too angry to speak.

'You should happy too, woman. She young, it good she find love, you want her to be alone forever?'

'Course not, but a foreigner? Them people never take Jamaican girls serious. He'll use her for a drugs mule. Use out her body and throw her to the wayside.'

'They not all like that, Miss Rootie, don't fry all

foreigners in the same fat. I come across many that are decent folks and he look like a sensible man to me.'

'You see him?'

'Yeah man! They make a handsome couple. I see the two of them at Meadows Inn.'

Ruthie's eyes grew huge with horror. 'In the guest house?'

'Yeah man! No need to fret, Miss Kat is a woman.'

She was fully aware of that. A grown woman capable of conceiving a child that would kill her. She didn't even know if Kat was taking precautions, she prayed she was but she couldn't be sure. Her child was wild, stubborn, unruly and followed her own heart.

'The guest house in the middle of town for de world to see and know! You think they... they... they doing any funny bizness—'

Old Man laughed, a bellowing laugh that shook his whole body, jerking his shoulders.

'Miss Rootie, of course! Young people are good at that, you don't 'member when you young and fruity?'

Ruthie blushed and turned away, fuming.

'It is the most natural thing, Miss Rootie, it keeps the heart pounding. Passion is good for the soul, a God given gift. You should try it,' he teased.

'Don't take serious things make joke, Old Man, it is a serious matter. He break her heart. She crying all day in the room and I don't even know what he did her. She won't talk. I only hope she take caution. If she take with child, it will kill her! Nellie Potato already smiling like Satan with a lost soul at the news of Kat with a beau... plus she see them on the beach last night arguing and now Kat crying like she been orphaned.'

'Don't fret too much. Young people always arguing cause them love the making-up afterwards.' He laughed cheekily.

Miss Ruthie became livid. 'Don't joke with me, Old Man; I want to phone Columbus to come back. Maybe he can put a stop to this.'

'Columbus couldn't put a stop to a push cart. You need to stop complaining about Kat and leave her to live some life.'

'I ever complain to you?' Her annoyance showed. She already regretted showing her vulnerability to Old Man, as she felt it might give him the audacity to voice his opinion more often.

'You is one miserable woman. You want to eat out at Sandy Tymes with me? I hear they doing cut price three course meal.'

Miss Ruthie negotiated this with her wiser self. If the meal was cut price and three courses, then it would not impede too much on Old Man's meagre wallet. She of course had to also consider the talk it would cause should anyone see her walking out with Old man, but at this moment she really didn't care. She needed the distraction from the fear that was forming in the pit of her stomach at the one word that kept popping up; pregnancy.

'Old Man, I accept your invitation,' she replied solemnly.

Fourteen
Ben

Ben could honestly say he was furious with Bubs. His innuendos had been as conspicuous as chicken pox and now Kat was hiding away. She hadn't been down to her usual spot on the beach and had switched off her phone. Bubs could be so insensitive at times and so infuriating.

'What were you attempting to do?' Ben fumed, slamming the door hard behind him. He had just returned from the beach in the hope of seeing Kat. He also knew he was being unreasonable to his friend; he knew he really should be thanking Bubs for forcing the situation to the fore. Kat needed to know the truth about him. But in that instance, sadness and pride was overpowering any common sense.

'Just to make you think, ain't no harm in that!' Bubs laughed lightly. He wasn't going to take Ben's anger seriously, not when Ben was in the wrong.

'Make me think? About what!' Frustration caused Ben's voice to shake.

'Claire, your daughters... remember them, India and Kenya?'

Ben slumped in the chair, words failing him.

'You don't understand,' was all he could muster.

'Oh yes I do, friend. I'm not your enemy; I've got your back. I'm not about to start telling you how to live your life but I want you to think about what you're doing. I think you've both been swept away and no proper thought is going into what's really going on. You have to see beyond this, when you go home.'

'It's my problem, Bubs, not yours. I made the decision to be with Kat.'

'To be with Kat? So, you're leaving Claire and the children?'

Ben glared at his friend. 'When did you become so fucking conscientious? How many women have you left holding your children?'

'Too many... but I'm not married, and I'm not you. Anyway, my meddling is done with; from now on I have nothing to say about your predicament.'

'First fucking sensible thing you've said.'

Bubs laughed, shaking his head in disbelief. 'What has happened to you, bro?'

'Katherine St Monica Lewis. She takes up as much of me as Claire and it feels crazy, thrilling and exciting, yet, daunting too. It scares me that I don't know how to control it.'

When he had married Claire, he never considered that another woman would be able to bring out such passion and intense feelings of, dare he say it, love. Yes. It was love. He loved her until it ached. It was a mad place to be. Her carefree, feel-the-fear-and-jump-anyway attitude had infected him.

Despite their differences, by the time Ben dropped

Bubs off at the airport the following afternoon, it was like nothing had happened between them. They were back to laughing, joking and slapping each other's backs. Bubs was as good as his words and mentioned no more about Kat.

'See you in London.' Bubs saluted and disappeared into the departure lounge.

Bubs's interference and mischievousness had been useful on one level. The guilt Ben had felt was no longer gnawing away, draining him like a parasite. It was all out in the open and it gave him the greatest sense of freedom. But that freedom came with a price: the void left by Kat. He called her mobile and left countless messages. In the afternoon, he took a stroll along the beach, and passed her empty throne. He was tempted to hop into a taxi, which he felt certain would know where she lived, but the look she had given him that last time he had seen her stalled his action. How could he leave Jamaica and not see her again? It was impossible to imagine.

He returned to the hotel and showered to the blaring reggae music on Irie FM. He then dressed in his Jamaican flag boxer shorts and a white string vest and settled on the balcony, a bottle of Red Stripe beer for company. Sunset was about an hour away—he could see which part of the Meadows was being rained on by the position of the large dark clouds.

Sunset came and left, and by then he was on his forth Red Stripe and hadn't eaten all day. His head began to feel light at the thought of spending another night without her. He was fast talking himself into doing something ridiculous, like taking the damn taxi to her house and shaking sense into her. He returned in the room to rub some repellent on, as the mosquitoes were beginning to annoy him and he had to keep slapping his arms and legs hoping to get one of the suckers.

He froze; he thought he heard a tap on the door and his name, said by the voice he could have picked out in a crowd.

'Ben.'

Kat was calling him. In two strides he flung the door open and she was standing there in a white dress, her hair free from its usual ponytail, falling curly, bushy and wild past her bare shoulders. It was a few more hesitant seconds before he dared to take her hand and lead her gently into the room. He smoothed back her hair, but it sprang back to chaos. It suited her, made her look love-swept and desirable.

'Sweet girl,' was all he could say.

*

They lay naked and tangled, arms and legs entwined beneath cotton sheets. She fingered the untidy tips of his braids absentmindedly.

'You dropped Bubs to the port?'

'Uh huh. He's got about five more hours of flight left. He'll be jet lagged for weeks, knowing Bubs.' He snuggled into the nape of her neck, inhaling her.

'Can you trust him?'

Ben knew exactly why she had asked that question. 'With my life.'

'No-one needs to be hurt.' Kat had spent hours working through his revelation.

It had knocked her out completely, leaving her feeling

confused and tearful and grief-filled. Mother Cynthy had said he held secrets, she just never expected it to be this. He was married. She had been through an internal battle. One voice told her to leave him, let him go back to his wife, the other asked her if she thought fate could make a mistake. Her head decided she would let him go; only her will and her heart differed. This debate with herself had led her back to his door.

Ben nodded in sincere agreement. 'I know. But you and me, we're more than any affair. I'm sorry I deceived you.'

'There are worse crimes than being married. I just never thought I would fall for anyone's husband. Miss Ruthie would die of shame... I don't even know how I'm going to handle this. Your deception hurts like hell.'

'Don't give up on me. I'm going to work something out.'

'What?'

'Let me buy you a house, we need time in our own space when I come to Jamaica, we're more than guest houses and hotels.'

'So, you want to make me a matey? A mistress?'

She felt him cringe. His voice was soft and pleading. 'I want you,' he pulled her close, 'let me have you.'

Kat felt her heart somersault; his words brought an intense heat to her body and a want so great that her eyes sprang tears. The pain was real and raw every time she thought of his wife, yet she could not muster the strength to walk away.

'You have me. What now? What will you do with me?'

'Love you.'

She sighed, her breath sounding tired, weary. 'My

friend Rosie says,' she turned her head to face him, 'that love as sweet as it is, cannot full a belly.' She used her forefinger to trace his eyebrows. 'And words do not have arms to hold you, to keep your company when it rains and your man isn't around.'

His silence was loud with anxiety.

'There's truth in Rosie's words. But just because you don't see me in front of you doesn't mean I'm not thinking about you or longing for you.' He hoped she wanted him as much as he did her. That she would give him the time to work something out.

'There's a lot to think about, Ben.'

'Of course,' he admitted with coyness. 'But we have only two days left.'

She undid herself from his arms and strolled across the room to pour a glass of water. He watched her naked form with his own inner thirst, the curve of her body enveloped by the sunbeam booming up from behind, painting her in splinters of light.

'You look like an angel.'

'Your mouth is sweeter than any mango I ever tasted.'

*

Two days flew by. Kat and Ben were inseparable. They enjoyed every second as if it was the last, knowing that the time would come when there would be an ocean between them. Their love was out in the open, she knew he loved her and she loved him and fate had done the rest. Of course she had her doubts, she couldn't shake the thought of his wife, and the fact that he was returning to her arms, but whenever she even entertained leaving him, her world crumbled. She surrendered to fate and the prediction; she would have Ben's baby.

It was an overcast day as Kat helped him pack in silence. He felt emotional as he fought to hold onto aspects of her, the slow smile that slid across her lips, the charcoal pupils that almost filled the whites of her eyes with the ability to conceal all emotions, her laughter, her banter and her intellect. He resisted the possibility that this could be the last time he ever saw her. It felt like she could read his mind as she clung to him, letting out gentle sobs.

'I've still got your shirt. And your sketch is finished, but I'll keep it so you have a reason to return.'

'I don't need that reason. I'll leave you my number. You have a mobile, please use it and keep it switched on, even when you get pissed with me. And when you agree, I'll pay for a landline.'

'Miss Ruthie won't hear about a phone in her house. She thinks it's a device of Satan and the CIA because Nellie Potato from the post office uses it to seep gossip.'

'Carry your mobile everywhere, keep it near you. That way we can keep in touch regularly. It'll be cheaper for me to do the calling, or I can send you some credit. I'll call you every day.'

'I can afford credit on a phone, we don't reach that poor yet. You guys in England have a really weird view of us. Not all Jamaicans beg for a living, you know. And every day may be a little exhausting.'

'I didn't mean to offend you.'

'I'm not offended. I just don't want you thinking you can buy me.'

'Must you always be so stubborn?' he said with a smile.

'It was predicted for me before conception.'

His face expressed misery. 'I miss you already.'

'When will you be back?' she asked, trying to conceal her own anguish.

'I don't know.'

'That's not an answer.'

He sat on the bed watching her with a mixture of desire and bleakness. She was always so to the point but he knew she was right.

'I still don't understand what's happened to me, but I know I want you.'

Kat sat on his lap with an arm around his shoulders. She had the edge on this. She knew why they had to meet; he had no idea that they shared destinies.

'We have something magical.'

He understood. He felt it. 'You're a witch,' he teased, 'you've bewitched me.'

She cupped his face with both hands and studied him. Ben felt like a creature under a scientist's microscope. She spoke with a caress in her voice.

'No matter what the outcome of "us" is, remember it was our fate.'

She placed her forehead on his, their noses almost touching, their lips but a breath apart. 'Mother Cynthy predicted you'd come and you came. She's never wrong about things. She also predicted something else, but I'll tell you about that another time. '

'You intrigue me.' He moved his lips even closer to hers.

'There will be karma for this, we got to know that.'

'Karma?'

'Yes, do you know what—'

'I know what karma is; I just don't know if I believe in it. I mean, what has an innocent child done to deserve some of the atrocities we see happen? Karma doesn't explain that.'

'No,' she spoke slowly, 'but just because you don't understand it, it doesn't mean karma isn't real.'

'I'll take my chances with you Katherine St Monica Lewis. Right now all that matters is that I can hold you, feel you, see you, because I know this time tomorrow my body will be London bound, but my heart will be here with you in Jamaica.'

Fifteen
Kat

Late Sunday morning Kat sat in her favourite chair on the small veranda eagerly awaiting Columbus, who had recently arrived back from Paris. Her toes curled with the anticipation of seeing him, her dear friend. They had met on her eighteenth birthday. He had been new to the Meadows, spending much of his time in the caves in the hills, chipping away at rocks, then taking pictures of the disorder he created. Folks called him the mad foreigner because he objected so adamantly to being called 'the English' or even worse, 'the Irish.' Nellie Potato had been first to call him Irish. She said it was because her aunt knew an Irish man who had pale skin that would burn and never tan, and red hair and moles scattered over his face, arms and shoulders, just like Columbus. Columbus was immediate in his corrections. He was French and his skin did not have moles, but *taches de rousseur*—freckles.

Columbus was always vocal in explaining his heritage. His mother was from a wealthy French family and his father a Scottish luxury car millionaire. After their divorce he had grown up between France and Scotland, spending his summer holidays with his father in Edinburgh, learning about the car industry but lived in Paris with his mother learning about marketing and sales for the family perfume business. He had been pulled apart by his parents his entire life, and it was only in the Meadows that he found an outlet for his love of archaeology, and a friend to share that with in Kat.

It was Old Man Jaguar who brought him along to celebrate Kat's birthday, belly full of rum and trying to impress Miss Ruthie with his new young foreign friend. Old Man had boasted of the wealth of the 'foreign man' who paid him more money for one day's guide into the hills than he made the whole week as a beach attendant. It goes without saying that Miss Ruthie was far from impressed with a young foreigner who wasted precious time and good money playing mud games in caves. She was initially against the friendship that started that day between Kat and Columbus, but eventually warmed to him after the obvious change in her child; he had a calming effect on Kat and her sickle attacks dwindled considerably. At first she thought it may have something to do with the daily and nightly prayers she offered up to her beloved Lord and Mother Cynthy's medicines and bush baths. But the small thought also niggled like an irritating mosquito bite that it could have something to do with Columbus' presence in Kat's life.

Within weeks of meeting Columbus, Kat knew she would never fall in love with him in the way he wanted and he was not the man from across the ocean Mother Cynthy predicted. They were comfortable with each other, which sparked rumours in the Meadows but she never cared about those, unlike her mother.

Kat loved the way Columbus would speak to her in French before repeating the sentence in English. The gesticulation whenever he spoke had initially made her laugh and think him rather eccentric, but quickly became one of the things she was most fond of. He was an only soul, just like her, an only child of aging parents and his mother, like Miss Ruthie, was lovingly overbearing and has dreams of him taking over the family business. His name had intrigued her, it belonged to a pirate, and she said as much when they met.

'My mother gave me my name... she said Columbus sounded like an aristocrat's son, which would make good for a successful business man. Can you imagine how she feels let down every time she looks at me?'

They had both laughed and Kat told him his mother was way off the mark. They shared similar appreciations; the universe, rivers, trees, plant life and the possibilities of the impossible. Over the years the friendship they started with deepened. Without changing direction into passion or love, it quietly extended its roots deeper into friendship, orchestrated by Kat who could never keep a straight face at the faint hint of Columbus trying to romantically entice her. Eventually he had stopped his efforts.

She had much she wanted to tell Columbus. To share with him what she so far had had to keep to herself. She checked her watch. It would be 5pm in England now and she wondered what Ben was doing. Ever since he left two months earlier she checked the time persistently, despite the fact that he called her daily.

She heard the old jeep's engine long before it pulled up. Samson sat by the gate expectantly as he did whenever

Columbus was near. She beamed as her dear friend jumped the gate like a prized racing horse and took the squeaky steps two at a time to swoop her into his arms. She clung to him, realising she missed him far more this time than any other. After Ben left she suddenly realised how empty her life had been.

'How have you been *ma chérie? Ca va?*' His warm hands cupped her face as he placed a kiss on each cheek.

Columbus was tall and slim with long sandy-red hair always in one untidy plait, and his round spectacles just didn't sit right on his narrow nose, which meant he had the habit of always adjusting them with his index finger.

'I'm alright. I missed you though. Let's go for a drive, I have so much to tell you.'

They drove to Rising River, where Columbus parked his jeep at the bottom of the hill and they strolled down to the river. He bought two cups of red pea soup. They wandered over to sit on the bridge by the river bank. The last time she had visited this place had been with Ben, she thought with a sigh. She gave to the river a sea shell; Columbus threw a piece of coral.

'It is raining back in the Meadows, look at that dark cloud over there,' he pointed.

'We have a couple of hours before it reaches us.' Kat broke from sipping her soup.

'We'll get back soon. Miss Ruthie will never forgive me if I let you get soaked. *Comment vas-tu vraiment, Kat?* How have you been? *Tu sembles fatiguée...* you seem tired.' He reached out to stroke her cheek.

'I'm tired but I've never been so happy in my life. I can't keep this up. I have to tell you my good news now... I've been busting to share it with someone.'

'*Quoi*? What?' Columbus laughed, his blue eyes holding her. She always had so much to tell after his return, and he always looked forward to hearing her take on the locals antics, and her impersonations of Miss Ruthie, Old Man and Nellie Potato.

'Swear you won't utter a word to a soul?'

'*Je te le jure...* I swear.'

'Swear on your life,' she insisted.

'I promise.' His smile was curious.

'I'm eight weeks pregnant.'

There had been no greater silence. She saw the blood drain from his face, confusion replacing the curiosity that moments ago appeared friendly. Try as she might she could not conceal her joy. How could she when her dream, the prediction Mother Cynthy made all those years ago had now come to pass. She was going to become a mother at last.

'You are what?' he spoke in a robotic tone. 'If I heard you correct, then you should not be smiling. Pregnancy in your fragile condition means disaster... *tu pourrais mourir...* you could die!' Columbus now looked at her smiling face in utter dismay. 'What have you done?' His outstretched arms, palms up and bent at the elbow, shook.

Kat knew the extent of his disappointment, his deep pain, but she could not sympathise, as this was what she had wanted, waited for. 'Be happy for me, Col. The doctors are not overly concerned about this. I can't live off Miss Ruthie's fear. Pregnancy won't kill me. That fear was passed on because my aunt Doris died in child birth, and she was a sickler. Things are different now. Just be happy for me,' she pleaded.

She saw his jealousy, even if they were not a couple, not lovers, but everyone thought they were and he had gained respect from the local men because of it. The hurricane raging in his thoughts was visible on his face as his arms flapped around like a mother hen returning to an empty nest. He stood angrily to his feet and walked away from her. For a long moment his back was turned, trying to assemble some logic to his thoughts, to her action.

'Be happy for you? How can I? You can be so impulsive, Kat.'

She wasn't going to apologise for it. 'It was my choice.'

Turning to her he spoke in a grim voice. '*Ma chérie*, you cannot have a baby; you know what Miss Ruthie says.'

'Yes, and you and I know Miss Ruthie is not a doctor, so don't try that... she's led by her fears and I won't be,' she spoke buoyantly.

'I take it Miss Ruthie does not know.'

'God no! No-one knows... only you, Paula, Rosie and Mother Cynthy so far.'

'Paula! Rosie! Mother Cynthy? You tell them before you tell me?' He thumped his chest so hard it sounded like a heavy thud, like someone had fallen from a great height onto the floor.

'Oh Col, you can be so dramatic. It was Mother Cynthy who told me, I didn't have to say anything. And Paula is a friend I can trust, so of course I'm going to tell her and Rosie,' Kat retorted. It annoyed her that Columbus could sometimes be so possessive.

'Mother Cynthy's prediction came true. You know

she predicted I would have a child... and with a man from across the sea.'

'I know you believe that but it does not make it true. And what about the father? Does he know?'

'Not yet.'

'Does he know about your illness?'

'Lord no! I don't want him to view me different.'

'Where does he live?'

'London. He was here for a break after working in Kingston. He's in real estate. There's no need for him to know right now. I-I have to sort things out in my head first.'

Columbus had his back turned looking into the river.

'River life is so noisy,' he spoke like someone hypnotised. 'Right now I can hear every swish of the fish's tails and sense every ripple of the water.' He turned and faced her in desperation, his fingers and thumbs pressed together and shaking.

'Kat, you have to face reality. You can get too caught in your own world. Once an idea forms in your stubborn head, it quickly hardens like rock. Your hardened thoughts become impermeable. They allow no outside interference or influence... *oui j'ai très peur pour toi.* I fear for you.'

A storm raged in her eyes but he continued, 'Kat, where are your senses, *ma chérie*. What on earth were you thinking?'

'I've been thinking about having a baby forever!' she blazed. 'And since I turned twenty-eight the thoughts come more often and stronger. I was thinking that maybe the Lord wants me to have my baby. I want to feel life move in me. I want to grow fat and vomit and complain about my ailments and have cravings for sardines and guava jelly. I can't wait to see the stretch marks running like car tracks down my belly. I was thinking that more than anything in this world, more than I want to live. I want a baby, Col, I want this baby.' She laid her hands on her still flat stomach.

Columbus exhaled in defeat.

'Miss Ruthie will die, you know that.'

Her lips gave way to a small smile and she spoke softly, 'She'll live forever; she just pretends to be mortal.'

They didn't come home until after sunset. Kat knew Columbus still had many unanswered questions. It was obvious he wanted to know a great deal more about Ben. But she was not willing to talk; she knew that her words would only shred his heart more than it did now.

'You know I have to blot out the images of your intimacy with another man; more intimate than we have ever been, will ever be,' he whispered so dejectedly that she turned and hugged him.

'You're still my dear friend, that won't change.'

Miss Ruthie sat in her rocking chair on the veranda, her paper bag of uncooked rice resting on her lap. Columbus waved to her from the car, turning down Kat's invitation to eat with them.

'It looks like the rain passed, the skies are clear again,' said Kat, feeling at peace. Sharing the news with Columbus had made it more real—she was going to be a mother. She would soon hold her very own baby in her arms.

'When will you tell her?' asked Columbus, staring intently at his friend.

She looked towards Miss Ruthie and suddenly felt sadness at how she knew her mother would react to her wonderful news. 'Not until she sees for herself. I'm going to pick up the iron and folic acid from the pharmacy. I don't want to see Dr Mattie because she'll just tell Miss Ruthie everything and all the pressure will be on.'

'Are you sure about… the baby, Kat?'

'Never been more sure of anything in my life.'

Over the following weeks, no greater joy was felt by Kat than when she thought of the baby growing inside her. She hid the books and pamphlets the doctor gave her under her mattress and only in the stillness of the night, when the soft snoring of Miss Ruthie drifted into her room would she take them out. Then she would read hungrily every detail and marvel at the pictures of the miracle forming within her.

Sixteen

Ben

London

Ben opened his eyes for the fifth time in an hour, and it was still only 6am on Saturday morning. Saturdays were always chill till noon time, unless business interrupted this flow. He knew he had a couple of hours before the children would come crashing in, and he really did need the sleep, but he no longer heard his own voice. Kat was now the voice in his head and he woke each morning itching to phone her, to hear the Jamaican melody floating down the ear piece. He missed the tropical sea breeze that explored and intoxicated him; the luscious green of the island that seduced and warped his senses and rendered him truly infatuated. The lifeless London summer skies could not compare. And most of all, he missed his new love.

He felt the movement of his wife easing her way into his arms, her head resting on his chest. He started stroking her back, as his body reacted to her warm softness.

'Morning, Benny.' Her sleepy voice was relaxed and happy. 'This feels so good, having you home. I never want to be without you again.'

He squeezed her tightly to him. 'And there was me thinking to go away more often because I've been back six weeks and each night the welcoming home from work is first class.'

She giggled, lazily crawling on top of him to pin him down beneath her. He looked up at her beautiful face; soft caramel skin and flushed, her soft brown curls tumbling way past her shoulders, her slanted eyes filled with adoration. She smiled, revealing a mouth full of perfect, even white teeth.

'I just want to make it much harder for you to ever be away from us for so long again. It was torture, Benny, fucking torture.'

Guilt flooded him and he knew he had to find a place to put moments like these; the ones that split him in two because for all the love he had for his wife, Kat loomed large in the background, too large to ignore. Before the guilt could take hold fully, he devoured her, losing himself in the familiar and delicious love which was theirs.

'It just amazes me how fast children change,' Ben said, reflectively, after their brief and passionate love making, before the children could wake. 'I missed you guys, like crazy.'

'And you noticed your eldest is developing breasts.'

'No she's not... they're just bed bug bites or something, we'll buy her a new mattress. My little girl is not growing breasts at eleven years old, for God's sake. I was just changing her nappies the other day.'

Claire laughed, running a hand over his braided head. 'You're broody; you want to try for that baby boy we're always planning? We shouldn't leave it too long, I'm thirty-three next birthday and they say by thirty-five a woman's eggs start to lose quality. Plus, remember I only have one tube.'

Ben hugged her, remembering the devastation after her ectopic pregnancy three years earlier. 'Don't worry, if it's our fate, we'll have our son, and if it's not, we already have two beautiful daughters.'

Cradled in his arms, Claire brought his face closer. 'I'm the luckiest woman in this entire world, to have a hubby like you. Look at you, going all fucking philosophical on me—talking about fate.' She kissed him. 'But you've been in a world of your own lately. Yesterday over dinner I called you three times before I registered to you.' And again the guilt knocked. Kat.

'Sweet girl, how about I treat you today. What do you want to do? Spend the day with Helen and the girls? Go shopping? What about your spa specials? Or what about me and you get loved up tonight at Crazy Bear, forget we've got kids.'

Her face broke into a tender smile. 'I'm definitely taking a rain check on that. But today I'm chairing the meeting at the Women's Forum, we're organising a Lupus fundraiser bake off, from 4 to 6pm. By that time you'll have picked up India from horse riding and Kenya from Saturday School.'

He gave a gentle sigh, placing a kiss on the top of her head. Things were back to normal.

Late afternoon, after Claire had gone and the children were out fulfilling their social diary, Ben sat in his study with the door closed and phoned Kat.

'You miss me?' he asked.

'Do you miss me?' she asked back.

'Yes. I miss watching the sunrise and the sunset with you. The beach and the river, all the things and places you took me to. The food and Ras Solomon's red pea soup.'

He heard her great laugh and he joined in, his heart expanding with joy.

'What are you doing today? I like to see you in my mind's eye and imagine you.' Her voice was soft and wistful.

'Well, it's Saturday and the girls are out, horse riding and Saturday School. Tomorrow I'll take them ice skating as I've been promising them ever since I came home.'

'Sounds amazing, ice skating. I still wonder how you can live in a country that is cold like an ice box. Miss Ruthie says it's sheer lunacy, people living in the cold, but I must admit the pictures I've seen of snow are beautiful. And I've seen that you have vast greenery in some parts of England.'

'Of course. It isn't cold all the time, so okay our seasons are unpredictable, but we do get some sunshine you know. It's June now, summer and no it's not hot like the Meadows, but it was fairly warm yesterday, I took the girls for an evening ride on their bikes.'

'You're a good father.'

'Thank you, I try,' he laughed.

'Your life must be so busy, work, the children... other commitments; you hardly have time to consider me.'

'Sweet girl, are you crazy? My thoughts are wrapped so tightly around you I wonder how you breathe.'

He heard her laugh, light and unfettered. 'I'm so

happy, Ben, although I'm still confused, but now I feel–I feel I have hope… and I have you to look forward to. I will see you again, won't I?'

His voice was thick with passion. 'How can you ask such a question? Of course you'll see me again. You're in me, my head, heart; you're in my blood, Kat.'

'So what exactly does that mean?'

He was quiet briefly, then he responded with what he hoped was conviction, 'You're my love.' The phone was pressed close to his ear because it was important that he could pick up any change in her breath, in her tones or sighs.

Her sigh was soft. 'Catch up soon.'

'Could be sooner than you think, I may have to come out there to close of business with the realtors, I'll let you know.'

Three days later, and a day before her Lupus bake off charity fundraiser, and just as Ben had come out of the shower, he came face to face with Claire.

'Ben.' Claire's face was pale and her long hair a wavy mess, he could see something wasn't right. She was clutching her stomach in pain. Ben quickly reached for her.

'What's wrong?'

'I–I–I don't know. It hurts like fuck, I…' She flopped in his arms.

'Auntie Joan,' he yelled, sweeping Claire into his arms and laying her down on the bed, touching her forehead, placing a finger under her nose to check if she was breathing. 'Auntie Joan, call an ambulance! Claire's passed out, something's wrong, hurry!'

He drove in the ambulance, holding her unresponsive hand until he had to let go so the Paramedics could do what they were doing. He wouldn't forgive himself if anything happened to her.

When they arrived at the hospital, a team of doctors were waiting to rush her away, leaving him alone with even more guilt. He had been looking forward to flying out to Miami to meet with a group of property developers, guest speakers at their annual property seminar. He had then planned to take the two-hour flight from there and hop over to Jamaica to see Kat before flying home. But now disaster had struck. Claire-Louise. What was he thinking? Was this karma? He sat down heavily on a chair in the waiting room, praying his wife would pull through.

Dr Scott approached him over four hours later and Ben sat routed unwilling to read the look on the surgeon's face.

'Mr Benjamin, your wife has had an ectopic pregnancy.'

Ben looked puzzled. 'A what? Are you sure? We didn't know, I mean I didn't know. She's pregnant?' He knew Claire wanted another baby, of course they were just talking about it the other day, but nothing was planned.

'She would have been had the egg not embedded in the tube. I'm sorry but we had to remove the tube.'

'But that's the second,' Ben said, looking pained. 'This will devastate her.'

'I'm sorry. You'll both need time, Mr Benjamin.'

'She had dreams for a son, a baby boy. Can we ever have a baby?'

Dr Scott nodded. 'This can be discussed later. Your

wife will make a full recovery. She's in post op right now, you can come back this evening, she'll be awake then.'

Ben walked out mechanically and was startled by the coldness of the July air. He didn't have a jacket on, as he had just rushed out behind the paramedics taking his wife into the ambulance. He signalled a black taxi and jumped in. He needed to get home to the girls, let them know their mother was alright. He had seen them coming down the stairs as he was leaving, heard India call him but he didn't have the time to respond. The news that her second tube had been removed would devastate Claire, but at least she was alive. Slowly he started feeling relieved. Claire would be okay. Karma was not involved in this.

Later that evening, when the hospital was busy with relatives and friends visiting, Ben arrived, an enormous bouquet of yellow roses—Claire's favourites, in his arms. He had thought of introducing 'baby's breath' to her but knew she might just be upset about the name at such a time. He walked apprehensively down the white-walled corridor; he hadn't noticed all these details earlier when Claire had been rushed in. He took a deep breath before coming in the room, where his wife lay still in a bed.

'Hi, sweet girl, how's the pain?' Ben lowered his head to place a soft kiss on her cheek, then laid the roses on the table beside the bed.

'It's awful, seems worse than the first time.' Her hand reached out and touched the roses.

'The doctor says you can come home by the end of the week. No sign of infection, you'll be fighting fit in no time.'

'I guess.'

'Claire, I'm here with you and we will get over this.'

'I know. I'm grateful to be alive, right? I'm alive.'

Quite unexpectedly she burst into tears. 'Oh Benny, I'm sorry. What am I going to do about the Man U kit? The one sitting in the cupboard for our son.' Her sadness moved him close to tears.

He stroked her hair and she held on to him, pouring her heart out through tears.

'The doctor mentioned IVF, but it's too much Benny, too much. I wanted another child, a son, but I can't—I, I've had two children and as many miscarriages and now a second ectopic, it's too much—'

'It's okay, there's no pressure here. Let me brush your hair?' he said with a shaky smile. She handed him the brush. 'And just you listen here,' he warned jokingly, the brush pointing in her face, 'any son of mine would have to be kitted out in an Arsenal kit, so forget about your Man U, girl.'

When he first met Claire-Louise it was apparent that she was an organiser of everything. She had the sparkling, bubbly confidence of a team leader with a link to anyone who was anyone. He had first encountered her at the Cherry Grove, an up-market Chelsea club Bubs had convinced him to tag along to, and it just so happened it was one of her Ladies Who Dance Nights. She was sitting at the bar when his eyes met hers, and he was instantly glad he had come. He sat on the bar stool beside her, noticing how well put together she was. Her jewellery was light, a gold bracelet, a white gold watch and what looked like a diamond ring on her middle finger. Her brown hair had blond streaked highlights, salon finished, he guessed, but her make-up was sparse and natural looking.

'Hi, I'm Ben, and you are?' he smiled politely.

'I'm kind of a brand ambassador,' she introduced herself. 'Claire-Louise Hall.'

'Kind of? What exactly is that, Claire-Louise Hall?' He couldn't stop grinning, her mannerism of explaining everything with a flip of her slender, well-manicured hand was endearing to him.

'I'm hired by Lupus Aware to promote their brand and help them increase their brand awareness, and of course raise funds.'

'I see,' Ben said dubiously.

'You do know what Lupus is, right?'

'Wrong... but I'm sure you'll tell me.'

'You bet your balls. I'll do more than that; I'll let you buy some raffle tickets for our annual summer dance. There's a TV up for prize as well, we really need the money.'

'He already has a TV,' Bubs interrupted from over Ben's shoulder. 'And you leave his balls right there in his pants.' He sat down beside her, facing Ben.

'Oh fuck!' she responded, eyeing Bubs with blatant disapproval and flicking her hair. She gave her back to him and spoke directly to Ben, 'Does he always speak for you, or can you speak for yourself?'

'Only when I let him,' Bubs quipped, grinning at Ben. Ben could see Bubs' sense of humour was nothing more than irritating to her.

'You need to forgive my friend; his sense of humour comes without brakes.'

She looked doubtfully at Ben. 'Sense of humour? Is that what it is?'

Before Bubs could respond again, Ben offered to buy her a drink, which she swiftly accepted, after which they found a quiet table in the corner to continue their talk.

That night she told him everything there was to know about her with great pride. Her mother, Jolene was a half Jamaican-Chinese teacher who gave up her career to nurture her three British-born children. She never had to work because her husband, who was Cuban and a lover of Castro, was a successful Harley Street dentist.

Ben listened, riveted. He was lost in her beauty, and found her warm and appealing, leading him to invite her out to dinner the following evening. She was unashamedly a twenty-first century girl, a designer-lover-girl and mouthy with it, but she had this big heart and gave many hours to the charity that touched her most. She was also a family girl, who saw children as a big part of her future, which made her even more attractive.

They married eighteen months later, after Claire became pregnant with India. It was another six years and two miscarriages before Kenya, their second girl was born.

Ben pulled up a chair close to her bed and sat down, placing the brush on the corner unit.

'Your mother called, she's on her way. Oh yes, she's still wondering after all these years why we called our children India and Kenya, after countries that are so impoverished.'

Claire giggled through her tears as he had hoped she would.

'Mummy can be such a goose, and you know she

just can't forgive you for not choosing the names she suggested.'

Ben shook his head. 'Name my children Elizabeth and Margaret, after the Queen and her sister? I think not! She took some getting used to, your mother, but I'm over Her Majesty Queen Jolene the 1st now.'

'You okay about this, Benny? Really okay?' she asked, frowning.

'Of course.' He stood up and perched on the side of the bed and briefly pecked her lips. 'Having a son isn't everything. I still have my girls, and we have each other.'

'I wasn't talking about the baby... it's just ever since you came back from Jamaica you've been distant. Are you glad to be home?'

Ben leaned forward and kissed her mouth with more feelings. 'Of course. I missed you all,' he said.

Claire was home from the hospital an hour when her first visitor arrived, the familiar three rings of the bell in quick succession her best friend Helen's signature ring.

'Benny, get the door. It's Helen,' she said from the sofa in the living room, propped up against cushions, her legs draped with a soft purple mohair blanket. She was absorbed in reading *Marie Claire* magazine, and looked up to see why he was taking so long to move.

Ben took his time finishing the sentence he was reading in the *Times* newspaper before answering the incessant ring of the doorbell. Helen breezed in carrying a money tree plant, which she promptly placed in Ben's arms.

'Hi, sweetie-pie!' she offered him a cheek, which he hesitantly touched with the side of his face. 'Is the sick lady alright?' She strutted down the hall way without waiting for an answer, her tall slender frame and long legs imitating a catwalk model. Her hair was a halo of tight, tidy curls with streaks of purple, which framed her slim face and her smile was wide, dazzling and practiced. Ben followed her into the lounge.

'Hello, girl! God you look awful!' Helen snatched the magazine and hugged her friend sympathetically.

Claire-Louise smiled. 'I'm just tired; I can't wait to hit the gym to increase my energy. Benny and the doctor want me to wait for eight fucking weeks!'

'Girl, I don't envy you.' Helen put on her exaggerated American accent, which comes and goes at her will.

'Thanks,' Claire sniffed.

'Oh Claire-Lou, look at your hair, what a mess! I'll do something with it, I'll do your nails as well, that'll cheer you up.'

Ben placed the tree on the coffee table in the middle of the room. He gave Claire a look of sheer exasperation.

'Oh Benny, sweetie-pie, can you get me a drink... make it something strong... brandy,' Helen continued, not bothered in the least by his expression of annoyance. Ben exited the room, mumbling under his breath about manners taking you far. He returned with the glass.

'Your majesty,' he mimicked a curtsey as he handed Helen the beverage.

'Thanks lots, honey-bun. Now how was Jamaica? Haven't really seen you to talk about your time there. Any handsome rich guys needing good loving?'

'There were plenty I'm sure, but none I came across were that desperate.'

She threw him a look of distaste. 'Ha! Ha! Ha! You are

so funny! Isn't your hubby funny, Claire-Lou?' She nudged Claire with her elbow. 'How about you, Benny? Any of them Jamaican girls groped your balls?' She laughed at her own joke and was quick to see the discomfort her humour caused. 'Sweetie-pie, I do hope I've caused you extreme embarrassment,' she teased, laughing. Claire covered her mouth to mask the amused smile.

'Sweet girl, I'm popping out to see Bubs,' Ben spoke directly to Claire. 'Auntie Joan will pick up the girls, I'll see you later.' He hurried out the room, but still managed to overhear them before closing the door.

'Actually you're quite fortunate he didn't stray during his time away. Most men do. Can you imagine Benny having an affair?'

Both women laughed at the absurdity of the thought.

Seventeen
Miss Ruthie
Jamaica

'Hard as nails. Hard as nails. Once she get a thought in her head there's no way in God's world will she change it.' Miss Ruthie sat in the white-walled sterile hall of the private hospital, her tear-lined face etched with grief, her red-rimmed eyes filling with more tears. Columbus sat silently beside her, sympathising with her dilemma and feeling the real fear of losing his friend.

'She would have gone the whole nine months without telling me... me, her mother,' Ruthie spat angrily. 'She tell you that she waiting till I see... well she nearly made it. How pregnant you say she is, four months?'

He nodded, staring down at the floor.

Miss Ruthie's voice still held disbelief. 'I should have known, she spending all them hours in guest house with that man, but I neva thought it would happen so soon. She didn't look any fatter... maybe her breast looked a little bigger, but I just neva thought she could be pregnant. I mean, she know she not strong and healthy, she know, so why she do such a thing? Why? And it happened so soon? She don't know the man long. It took me over twenty years to get pregnant and she, sick as she is does it in two weeks! Your purpose, Lord, I cannot see.'

Columbus could give the only answer Kat had given him: 'She wants a baby more than she wants to live. That is what she told me.'

'That don't make the slightest bit of sense.'

'Not to you, me or a lot of people, but to Kat it makes perfect sense.'

'And you know the father lives in foreign—Hingland?'

'Yes, she told me.'

'And you don't know him? Yet you live in Hingland half the year?' Her angry eyes mauled him.

'I live in Paris and I spend a few months in Scotland each year with my father, Miss Ruthie, and I do not know a lot of people in Scotland and even less in England, which is hundreds of miles away,' he defended.

'Oh, Sweet Jesus!' Miss Ruthie despaired, burying her face in her hands, rocking to and fro. She had hoped it was all over between Kat and the man after she spent the day in her room crying. They had obviously made up before the foreigner left. And now Kat was pregnant, keeping it a secret from her, and would have gone on doing so too, if not for her collapse on her secret weekly hospital visit. Her blood count was so low they admitted her immediately. She was in need of a blood transfusion. Now she lay hooked up to the damn machine which was pumping oxygenated blood around her frail body. Miss Ruthie begged God for forgiveness. She needed forgiveness because with all her heart she wanted the baby to die. That way she felt Kat would stand a chance of recovering.

'I always told myself that you and Kat would court one day. How could you make this man come between you?'

'There was nothing to come between, Miss Ruthie,' Columbus admitted sadly. 'Kat and I are friends. I wish she could love me the way I love her... she has always believed in the unbelievable, always. If you tell her it can't be done, she shows you how it can be done. Never a dull moment with her, even to sit in silence.'

'So you don't know this man?'

'How could I? He was here and I was in Paris. It is you who should know him.'

'Me?' Miss Ruthie spat, indignant. 'She takes them walks up to the beach everyday, I don't follow her! I neva know she was planning, scheming to have something that will kill her. I never once thought she could be serious about a foreigner. She's as hard as nails.'

Miss Ruthie stood shakily to her feet. Her lips trembled with a smile of relief as she saw Dr Mattie walking towards them.

'Oh Dr Mattie, you see what Kat do to herself? You see how foolish she is?' Miss Ruthie babbled as the doctor squeezed her hand.

'Wipe your tears, Miss Ruthie, I've examined her, she's stable, she's okay.'

'Can't they take that baby from her? It must be sucking her strength. Wouldn't she stand a better chance if it was gone?'

Doctor Mattie shook her head.

'The general opinion is that the pregnancy with sickle cell should be closely monitored, it's not necessarily a threat to life, Miss Ruthie. Sit down, let's talk.'

The doctor sat the other side of her. 'Kat was extremely anaemic, that's why she collapsed. She's made this choice Miss Ruthie, and we have to respect it and do everything we can to bring her and her baby through this.'

'But she will die,' Ruthie broke into a cry.

'She actually has a greater chance of surviving. She knows what she's on that hospital bed fighting for. She knows about the baby growing inside her and I think that alone if nothing else will pull her through this. If any complications develop later... decisions will have to be made, but until then...'

Ruthie sobbed inconsolably. 'With that tube going in and out of her; I can't see how she can survive delivering a baby.'

'I can't give any more assurance than what I've already said, presently continuing the pregnancy presents no risks. She can go home to take it easy for a few days. Just keep her well-fed and hydrated, she'll keep to her fortnightly antenatal checks and the medication.'

Once at home Miss Ruthie paced the veranda like a cat on a hot tin roof, delaying having to enter her empty house. The thought that Kat might never come home, might not survive the pregnancy struck such panic into her that she collapsed in her rocking chair, her head bowed sobbing and prayed, asking God to be merciful and to grant her child long life. She called on the spirit of her dead husband to oversee his offspring, to do all he could to prevent her from an early passing. She called out to her own mother and father, such was the grief that engulfed her.

'Miss Rootie, take heart, woman. Better must come,'

she heard a voice say through her sobs. 'God not taking you to no place he won't protect you... just take heart, be strong and hold tight.'

The voice was soft and warm, so familiar.

'Miss Rootie, you hearing me? You not alone, woman, you not alone.'

She stopped and looked up. The voice was so close, so real she felt as though it was right next to her.

'Old Man? It's you?'

Old Man Jaguar's face was a mash of concern, inches away from hers.

'Yes, Miss Rootie girl, I'm here right by you, I'm not leaving you alone.' His hand reached out and stroked her tears away. 'You're not alone.'

'Oh, Old Man, I'm so unhappy. I'm afraid Kat will die, and I'm so vex with her.'

She sobbed and leaned forward, burying her face into his chest as his arms pulled her closer.

'I'm right here with you, Miss Rootie, I'm right here.'

His arms were a comfort from the thoughts of losing her daughter. 'Oh, Old Man, Kat did something stupid—'

'Having a baby isn't stupid, Miss Rootie.'

Ruthie moved out of his arms. 'How you know Kat having baby?'

'Nellie Potato says her grandson's girlfriend having a baby and says Kat is in the same hospital—in maternity.'

Ruthie stood up with shaking clasped hands. 'Dear Lord! The whole Meadows knows now! The shame! The shame! Everyone will be asking about the father. Oh, the shame.'

Old Man stood up and took her hands. 'Listen to

you,' he chastised, 'ready to worry about what people think. Instead of worrying about them, let you and me pray for Kat.'

She blinked hard. 'You, pray? Do you even like our Lord Jesus? Do you know how to pray?'

'Just because I don't sit in church with your hypocrite friends every week doesn't mean I don't like Jesus, and yes, I know how to pray. I had to learn to ask the Lord how to get a stubborn woman like you to marry me.'

Together they closed their eyes and Miss Ruthie gratefully allowed Old Man to lead in the prayer for her daughter's life.

Eighteen

Jamaica

Kat

Columbus and Rosie collected Kat from hospital two days later. She was tired but looked happy and in good spirits. She sat in the passenger seat as Columbus drove the ten-mile journey back to the Meadows. The afternoon was fresh after the rain and she almost wished she didn't have to return to the Meadows' humid heat, or have to face Miss Ruthie. Her secret was out now for all in the Meadows to see, not that it bothered her but she knew it would her mother. The breeze was cool on her face and she opened the window further. As they drove, vendors at the side of the road waved their merchandise in the hope of a sale.

'Can we stop? I feel for some jackfruit.' She was glad she could finally boast to Rosie about her cravings.

'Those do not look fresh; we can stop nearer the Meadows,' Columbus spoke gently.

'I don't want to eat it; I just want to smell it.'

'Pregnant women do some strange things,' Rosie said. 'I 'member when I was carrying Simone, I would smell tar all day long.'

The jeep pulled up outside the gate, just as Miss Ruthie was sweeping the yard. She turned away as Columbus and Rosie assisted Kat out of the vehicle.

'Afternoon, Miss Ruthie,' Kat spoke cautiously. It was difficult trying to conceal her pleasure. She knew her defiance was clear, as she saw the despair on her mother's face.

Miss Ruthie did not respond. Instead she busied herself, seemingly too afraid to look at the pain that had become her daughter.

'Don't be vexed, Miss Ruthie,' Kat's words were loaded with a plea. Her mother looked at her like a stranger with the audacity to pass a personal comment.

'You young people nowadays really don't understand that actions have consequences, that you will surely reap what you sow.' She looked up to the heavens. 'I prayed to my Maker from the very depth of my soul, begging to be given the gift to understand you.'

Miss Ruthie leaned against the broom in her hand and looked wearily at Kat. 'I cannot remember ever wanting something so badly that I would risk my life for it. You know how I longed for a baby; I remember the feeling month after month when my blood came, but if I knew my life would end with a pregnancy—there's no way on God's earth or in his heavens would I do that.'

Kat knew it. She knew Miss Ruthie would have continued to take the scorn and the gossip from the town folks; what she would never have done is jeopardise her God-given life and couldn't forgive anyone who would.

'Your fear about Aunt Doris was put onto me, Miss Ruthie. I feel fine,' Kat insisted. 'I only passed out because my iron was low. I can do this. It's what women do every day and me being a sickler is not a death sentence.'

'Puss and dawg don't have the same luck!' Miss Ruthie spat.

'Dr Mattie says the baby and I are okay.'

'For how long? Your Aunt Doris died in child birth, and she was a whole heap stronger than you! How soon you forget things.'

'I don't forget, Miss Ruthie, but I can't live life fearing other people's experience will become mine.' Her voice shook and her nightmare that wrecked her sleep two nights earlier dared to flash its bright light. She had dreamt seeing a bubbling pond of fishes suffocating. What did it mean? Would she lose her baby?

Mother Cynthy's distinct figure appearing at the height of the afternoon was a welcomed sight for Kat. She went into her room and left the window open so that she would hear any complaints her mother had to make.

From her window she watched Cynthy make her way slowly up the wooden stairs to the veranda where Ruthie sat in her customary position, straw hat perched on immaculately groomed hair, her mouth crunching through uncooked rice. Kat didn't have to wait long before the conversation drifted towards her.

'Good Lord, Miss Rootie, give peace of mind a try! Your face looks like thunder at war.'

Ruthie made no attempt to adjust.

'I have to keep telling people that Kat alright. I don't give them no information about her pregnancy or father of the baby and all the things they want to know, I just tell them she's alright. I avoid Nellie Potato like a rattle snake. The poison that woman can wield is potent enough to destroy the Blue Mountains of Jamaica. Kat, pregnant for a foreigner! Her daddy, Glenrick Desmond Raymond Saul Joshua Lewis is turning in his grave.'

Words were not always necessary between Mother Cynthy and Ruthie, sometimes they would both sit for hours barely speaking, yet Kat felt a whole conversation had taken place. Mother Cynthy could see on Miss Ruthie's face the fear that consumed her.

'You have always paid too much mind to what people think, Miss Rootie.'

'I wish you did tell me 'bout Kat, Mother Cynthy, you knew all along and you neva even warn me.'

'How could I?' Cynthy placed her laden basket by the feet of the chair she sat in. 'When I get visions, I give it only to the persons involved, is not like Kat is a little child, she's a grown woman, Miss Rootie. I tell her and it up to her if she share it with anyone.'

'This is different, Cynthy! This is life or death! You should let me know.'

Mother Cynthy sighed. 'How is Kat?'

'She resting in her room with the infernal selfish phone.'

'It's a cellular phone, Miss Rootie, you talk of it like it's a tool of the devil.'

'It's a very selfish piece of equipment... she on it to that foreign man, day and night.'

'She's twenty-eight, Miss Rootie, she have to make her own choices and decisions. If you mus' know, the last thing she wanted was to worry you.'

'Yes, but she wanted the baby more! Who does she have to look after that child should something happen to her? I can't start with a baby at my age—she jus' never think sensibly and I can't forgive her.'

'Your lineage grows strong because of Kat. If she had no children, where would you and Glenrick be after her body leaves this earth? When our Lord Jesus Christ speak about eternal life, it's all about leaving pieces of ourselves behind. We live on through our children and their children. Glenrick would have wanted grandchildren, you know that!'

Miss Ruthie sighed and closed her eyes. She remembered in the hospital all those years ago, when Glenrick had held Kat in his arms and whispered in her tiny ears. She remembered him telling Kat to give her a grandson to play around her feet. Tears escaped through her closed eyes. 'Will... will she live, Mother Cynthy? Will she even live through this?'

'I see noting that tell me she won't... but only our Maker know for sure.'

*

Kat lay completely still in her bed, forming sleep in order to avoid any conversation with Miss Ruthie. The faint and distinct scent of ginger and mint lingered under her nose and created an urge to sip a cup of the steaming liquid. Before she moved to get up, a tightening, engorging feeling began spreading through her upper body. She felt it mostly in her chest. It was a new feeling, strange to her, but not frightening. She opened her eyes, staring up at her ceiling, the new white paint unable to completely hide the renovation so desperately needed. She looked down at her breast, enlarged by her pregnancy and saw her cotton night dress had two round patches of damp. Milk! Her breasts were leaking milk. Her stomach was still to show obvious signs that she was pregnant, but her breasts had. Suddenly she noticed her mobile was ringing, and grabbed it quickly.

'Hello, Ben,' she said, recognising his number.

'Hey, you, my sweet girl. I was beginning to think you'd thrown me away.'

'Nothing like that.' She was still feeling tired after her stay in hospital but she didn't want to alarm him with her news. She had so far not mentioned her pregnancy, as she didn't know how to or what to say.

'So, where were you? I wasn't getting through for a few days. Found another man? Got it together with Frenchy?'

She laughed weakly. 'No, we had a power cut and I couldn't charge my phone,' she lied but considered it far too small to be guilt-ridden by it. 'How have you been? How are the children? I dreamt you—'

'I've been dreaming about you too. I cannot keep it secret any longer: I'm coming to Jamaica.' His enthusiasm cut her short.

'When?' Panic sprang loose like a jack in the box. Fortunately for her Ben took it as excitement.

'Two weeks' time. Cracks have appeared in some of the houses in Kingston and my boss wants me to check it out.'

'How long will you be staying?' Kat ran her hand over her stomach. There was still no real sign that she was pregnant. Apart from her breasts, which had gone up a bra size, she fitted quite comfortably in her shorts and jeans, without any sign of the protruding abdomen she longed for.

'Four nights and five days, not long enough.' His

disappointment was solid. 'I want you to come stay with me in Kingston because I won't get the time to drive down to the Meadows. I'll send some money through Western Union for you to take a taxi. You're coming or I'll come for you myself!' His voice told her he would be taking no excuses. It was only five days. She could do five days, and she so longed for him, it ached.

'No need for that,' she chuckled, 'I'll even meet you off the plane if you like.'

'I'm coming in at Kingston Airport, arriving 3.20pm. I have a driver all set; I'll get him to pick you up first. Get the taxi to Kingston an hour earlier to meet him.'

'Okay. But please, no sending monies for taxi, I can afford to get myself to Kingston.'

'Still as stubborn as ever. I missed you, girl. Don't suppose you've lost any sleep over me? Most probably too busy painting or throwing gifts to the river goddess. Is she still stealing people's shoes? Is your best friend around?'

It pleased her that he remembered those things. It meant he thought about her with Columbus. He was jealous! She was elated.

They talked and laughed some more, making plans for when he would be in Jamaica before finally hanging up. Kat fell asleep with her phone clutched against her chest, smiling.

The intoxicating rush of desire she felt at the thought of seeing Ben again had to be concealed under the mundane. She kept to bed rest, religiously taking her medication and the herbal mixture Mother Cynthy had given her. She had two weeks to build her strength, and despite

Miss Ruthie's disapproval of the situation, she prepared healthy meals three times a day and insisted that Kat finished every morsel on the plate. Ras Solomon came a few times with a flask of red pea soup and Rosie made regular visits with bottles of spring water and peanut porridge, bringing the latest gossip and giving Kat what she so badly needed: laughter and the opportunity to revel in the coming baby.

The day Ben was due to arrive Kat got up extra early, when the sky was still pitch black and the chickens and Samson were stilled by sleep. She showered, packed and dressed all before Miss Ruthie could rise. She left a brief note saying she was going away for five days, not revealing her plans for those days even to Columbus. He would have become withdrawn and moody, a common trait since finding out about her relationship with Ben. She had not anticipated his reaction, or Miss Ruthie's. Miss Ruthie had become monosyllabic, looking at her with disgust and disappointment. Kat was not looking forward to them finding out about Ben being married.

She could count on one hand the number of times she had visited Kingston. She knew why. The heat was intense with far fewer trees to shade beneath, and no hint of the cooling sea breeze, it felt as though she had been put on a barbecue and was steadily roasting.

She arrived in Kingston around midday. The bus journey had been fraught with a series of stops to allow people to eat, ease their bladders, mend a punctured tire and stop a fight between a couple accusing each other of infidelity.

From the bus park she jumped into a taxi which

dropped her outside the guest house's huge bamboo gates where she was to meet Ben's driver. She wasn't due to meet him for two and a half hours, so she took out her pad and pencils and began tidying up his portrait. It was the first piece of work she completed with satisfaction and couldn't wait for him to see it.

The driver arrived right on schedule in his chauffeur's uniform and on the way to the airport the rain came as no surprise. Nowhere could there be such intense heat without Mother Nature intervening to balance the situation. The dried cracked earth drew the rain in like ink on blotting paper and the air smelled of wet earth and sour gutters. Kat wound up the window inside the taxi and asked for the air conditioning to be switched on. She was already missing the fresh air of the Meadows.

The rain had petered down to a fine drizzle as the driver, who had been mainly quiet on the journey, left her in the car while he went to meet Ben. She nearly jumped out of her seat at the sight of him, dressed in navy blue trousers and white shirt. His braids were neat, as if they had just been done. A pang pulled at her heart as she wondered if it was Claire-Louise who had done the braiding. If he had sat patiently between her thighs as she parted and plaited and they had laughed and joked with each other and maybe even ended up in bed.

'Hey you.' He climbed into the back seat beside her; his mouth was on hers before she could respond. She closed her eyes and savoured his moist, warm kisses. He sipped her lips like a chef tasting his creation, his tongue flicking in and out of her mouth.

'Missed you so,' he mumbled between mouthfuls.

'Me too,' she breathed.

The return journey to the guest house was far quicker but that could very well be the result of getting absolutely lost in pent-up desire and passion. It was only when the car came to a halt that she even remembered they weren't alone.

'Remember this?' She reached into her bag and pulled out a cardboard tube and handed it to him.

'A gift for me?' He smiled teasingly. He opened the tube to reveal her portrait of him. 'Wow! This is great! You wonderful woman, you!' He kissed her feverishly again. 'You have real talent, you're a true artist. Am I really this good looking?' He laughed, admiring the sketch of himself. 'This is amazing, you've even captured my untidy hair. I'll keep it forever! How much do I owe you?'

She thumped him playfully. 'This time it's for free.'

He objected strenuously, 'No way! We made a deal. You sketch and I'd pay, now how much? You were clear at the beginning that I would have to pay.'

'Pay me what you will.'

'Okay, give me your bank details and I'll arrange for that.'

The room was beautifully decorated with white sheets embroidered with gold thread and a plasma screen television occupied most of one wall. Beneath their feet a Persian mat made up of the colours of the rainbow, soft on marble flooring and a fridge stacked with drinks for every taste and as a special gift, mango ice cream.

Ben impatiently tore at her blouse. 'I want to see you naked, I want you now!'

Kat froze. She didn't want a close inspection that

could reveal her condition. She pulled in her stomach. He had two children so he must know what a pregnant woman looked and felt like. His lips travelling her neck towards her breasts was turning her knees fluid. Suddenly she didn't care. She had only five days of this and she didn't want to spoil it with any hang-ups. She didn't know when next she would see him and have his adoration like this.

'Look at you!' he enthused when he had peeled away all her clothing. 'You look like you've gained weight.'

The move to cover herself was automatic, but he caught her hands and held her at arm's length. 'Don't hide from me, that's so unlike you. I love your body. You just look different, more... womanly.'

He exhausted her. His passion came in floods and was consistent for hours. As darkness enveloped the room, he held her close and circled her breast, sensitive from the pregnancy and his hungry lips.

'Even your breasts are bigger,' he whispered in her ear. She said nothing, even when his fingers traced circles over her stomach outlining his baby. 'You look amazing, there's a glow to you, and no signs of missing me.'

'The glow came today,' she smiled. 'I couldn't wait to see you, to touch you, kiss you, love you. You've got me weak.'

'Good! I need you weak in my arms. How's Miss Ruthie?'

'She's her usual worrying self.'

'What's she got to worry about now?'

It crossed her mind to say something, to let him know about his child growing within her. It was still hard for her to believe she was pregnant and until she held that little bundle in her arms and knew she had a real baby, she could not chance telling him, just in case he didn't want this baby as much as she did, or worse still, in case he didn't want this baby at all. And just in case Miss Ruthie turned out to be right, in case her body really wasn't strong enough to carry her baby and she would succumb like Aunt Doris. She still feared that nightmare, the one with the suffocating fish, and her interpretation of it. She hadn't even told Mother Cynthy about this dream; as if holding it in will somehow prevent it from happening.

'Even if there's nothing to worry about, Miss Ruthie would create something.'

'She gave you problems to come to Kingston? Didn't she want to know who you were staying with?'

'I'm a grown woman. I didn't explain a thing. I left a note.'

'And what about your best friend? Mr Frenchy. Does he know about me?'

She couldn't help laughing. 'No need to worry about Col, I told him all about you.'

That answer seemed to make him happy.

'We have five days, what do you intend doing with me? Take me to some river who'll steal my shoes if I don't give it something? Or more chanting Rasta men who'll give me a lecture and a hard time? Perhaps a trip to the top of Meadow View to see the sunset?'

She knew strenuous activities were out. 'Let's just have some "us" time. I want to spend the four nights and five days in your arms. Soon you'll be gone again... back to your life.'

Ben stroked her hair. 'I'm working on this, Kat, I really am.'

The following morning they had breakfast by the pool under a huge umbrella. The sun was already ruthless and Ben dipped in the pool to keep cool. Kat watched him socialise with the other guests, all of them laying down or sitting up relaxed on floats. The smell of fried eggs, dumplings, and ackee and saltfish was thick in the air and as Kat munched on her last spoonful of fruits, her phone rang. She was relieved to see it was Rosie. Last night she had turned it on silent and seen that Columbus had called at least twelve times. She felt a pang of guilt not answering, but knew the tiresome alternative if she did.

'Kat! Where are you?' Rosie bellowed.

'What's the matter, Rosie? Why are you calling at this time of the morning, and shouting?'

She heard Rosie's heavy sigh. 'Because Columbus has just come calling at my blasted house looking for you! And him say Miss Rootie worried that you gone missing with you sick pregnant self. Where are you?'

Ben began calling her, waving for her to join him in the pool.

'I'm pregnant, not sick and I'm in Kingston... with Ben. I'll be home by the end of the week, and anyway, I left a note telling them I'd be away—I wish they'd stop treating me like a child.'

'Then you shouldn't act like one. Why you never just tell them the truth? Have you told Candy Eyes about the baby?' The disapproval rose high in Rosie's voice.

'No,' she lowered her voice to a whisper despite Ben being too far away to hear. 'He thinks I've put on weight, but he doesn't realise I'm pregnant.'

'Well, you don't look pregnant yet. Not like me. At three months I was already showing. This would be a good chance to tell him.'

'Kat!' Ben was waving at her.

'I've got to go Rosie, Ben wants me to join him in the pool. I'll see you when I get back.' Kat felt uneasy. She was holding back the truth about so many things but how, she argued with herself, could she tell Rosie, Miss Ruthie and Columbus that Ben was married and how could she tell Ben she was carrying his child?

'What you want me to tell Columbus? He knows I know more than I say, he'll be back again today, mark my word,' Rosie continued.

Kat didn't want to think about Columbus or Miss Ruthie until she had to.

'Oh, Rosie, tell them anything. I'm sure you can come up with something—'

Rosie sounded frustrated. 'Like what! Listen gyal, I don't want Miss Rootie blaming me for your actions. She already looks at me like I'm the one that bred you.'

Kat laughed. 'Don't mind her.'

Kat heard the hesitation at the end of the phone and knew Rosie had more to say.

'I hope Candy eyes is worth it, all this sneaking around... Why didn't he come back to the Meadows? You should have insisted he came. He should meet Miss Rootie; show her he's serious about you. I don't understand why you don't tell him about the baby... what future you going to have together when you hiding so much?'

Nineteen
Ben
London

Ben was dubious but he had to support his wife's moon gathering, as she called it. Claire, along with friends, was having a moon party. He had just returned from Jamaica a week ago and he had been struggling with the guilt of being with Kat and away from Claire. The guilt of being with Claire and away from Kat. It was guilt all round and he was drowning in it.

He was lying on the bed as she was getting ready and he watched her add make-up to her eyes, then apply lipstick and finally get the straightening comb to elongate her natural curls.

'So it's a moon party?'

'Yes, it's Ariel's idea, female power is more potent tonight.'

'And how can us males benefit from some of that potent power?' He smiled appreciatively at her appearance.

She viewed him wearily, sadly. He smiled gently, getting up off the bed and standing in front of her. 'I'm not rushing you, I wasn't trying it on. All in your time, okay?' He kissed her forehead and she put her arms around his waist, hugging him.

'Just be patient with me, you have been so far and I appreciate it. I just want to feel like myself again, you understand.'

'Yes. Of course.'

She stood on tip toes to kiss his lips. 'Make sure you listen, it's good for a man to get a glimpse of a woman's world.'

Ben made himself as scarce as Claire would allow and the children were staying with their grandparents for the weekend so he headed for his study, leaving the door ajar, wide enough so he could hear and partially see.

The party was a small gathering of women, six including Claire and Helen. Ben watched from the door as they came striding in. There was Portia, as loud as Helen but with more tact. Taylor, Miss I-have-it-all; Ariel, Miss I-lead-and-you-follow and Lorna, Miss don't-give-me-too-much-to-think-about. He hadn't hidden his opinion about Claire's friends from her. Claire was fully aware and had responded with, 'Do you really think having Bubs as a friend qualifies you to speak about my fucking friends?' He had laughed and made no further comment about them.

Auntie Joan provided big jugs of rum punch, bite size snacks as requested by Helen and the music volume was low to allow for conversation. With the easy flow of alcohol there was just raw, uncensored female talk. The conversation floated across the hall towards him.

'I think a woman must know and love any man she has sex with...' Lorna stated.

'And what century do you live in?' Helen rebuffed.

178

'I think Lorna has a point,' Ariel added. 'Sex has just been devalued by the media and so-called celebrities, social networks, it isn't sacred anymore.'

'Am I sitting among a bunch of nuns or what?' Helen splattered, reaching for her drink. 'Thank God sex ain't sacred, right... because if it were we might all have to be married to the first man we ever have sex with, forever. Now think before you answer, girls. Would you really want to be stuck forever with the first man you ever fucked?'

The room filled with laughter and voices tumbling over each other to answer. Ben couldn't hear anything clear, but he couldn't curtail the smile that curled his lips.

Taylor added her words of wisdom, 'I think it depends. Leon was my first, sixteen I was, and here we are twenty years later, married with three kids. It still feels good.'

'Leon was not your first,' Helen pointed out with a finger. 'You and that one with the bandy legs, what's his name again?' She looked at Claire for the reminder. 'You know, the one that use to play football for QPR reserves and had a sister that got pregnant in school.'

'Liam—'

'Liam, that's the one,' Helen cut Claire off.

'Actually Liam didn't finish the job...' Taylor corrected, 'he started but he said it was too hard. Said I was as tight as a chicken's arse and gave up.'

Their high-pitched squeals hit Ben's ears, but he couldn't help laughing either. In a strange way he felt privileged to be eavesdropping and having a wife who was okay with it.

'Okay girls, calm down, calm down,' Ariel giggled. 'We're supposed to have positivity fill the room on such a night, full moon, ladies—all power to us. Now let's get the ball rolling with the first game. Let's start by going around the room and each of us saying one positive thing about ourselves, using one word.'

'That's difficult for me,' Portia spoke for the first time. 'There are just too many positive things about me to try and keep it to one specific.'

Ariel gave her a friendly slap. 'Okay, I'll start. Dynamic.'

'You are so not,' Helen laughed.

'You don't get to be the judge here, Helen,' Ariel huffed. 'Next... Claire, your turn.'

Ben leaned forward in his chair, eager to hear his wife's response.

'Loyal,' she said simply.

Ben's heart sank. Loyal suited her.

'You're more than that,' Helen said, squirming. 'You can do better.'

Claire shrugged. 'I think loyal is one of the most awesome thing a woman can be. Especially when you have a family.'

They were all quiet for a beat.

'Well I for one agree,' Taylor piped in. 'I know I started having the children young, but Leon and I planned it. We thought it better to get it out the way during our twenties so that I could at least have a career, which I do,' she said proudly. 'But being loyal to each other is what keeps our marriage strong.'

'You can't say any different,' Lorna spoke fast. 'You've done fucked up your life, thirty-six with three kids, what else are you going to say?'

'What do you mean, fucked up my life?' Taylor demanded. 'My kids are the best thing to happen to me—they gave my life new directions and taught me so much. I was able to return to work, flexi-hours approved by my director. Having kids doesn't have to stop you, and I understand what Claire means. Loyal is an amazing, positive, awesome word.'

'That all said and done,' Helen chirped. 'I think this is a dumb, boring game... how about we talk sex, like has a man ever asked you to do something so nasty you wanted to kill the motherfucker?'

'Yes, you guys remember Dave,' Portia said, 'that owned the mechanic shop off the hill? Well you know we dated for about two months and I dropped him like hot iron. That's because he asked me if I'd let him watch another woman go down on me.'

'What the fuck is wrong with them men!' Helen shrieked. 'You should have told him to let you watch a man go down on him.'

'That's tame,' Lorna said in her laid-back way, 'the shit I can tell you would make you spew.'

Ben heard whispered responses his ears couldn't pick up and laughed lightly. Then Ariel said, 'Helen, is this the time and place to be talking sex... in Claire's house with you know who across the way.'

'What the fuck! You think Benny boy don't know about sex?'

'This always happens when Helen has more than three glasses of anything, she starts trouble,' Taylor laughed.

Ariel sounded slightly agitated, 'Okay... let's go back to positivity. If you were stuck on a desert island and could have one thing, only one thing, what would you want?'

'That's easy; I'd want a big, thick vibrator—' Helen started and was cut off immediately by Ariel, who asked, 'Thank you Helen, Portia?'

'Me, I'd want fresh water, you know being on an island you're surrounded by the salty sea and I wouldn't want to have to go searching, too much hassle.'

'I'd want cooked food,' Lorna ended.

Claire cleared her throat. 'Another chance... just want one more chance, that's all. I'm talking chances.' She coughed. 'I'm aware that I'm a little heavy with alcohol, and my emotions are bubbling to the brim, but I feel I have to get this feeling out before it explodes, fucking killing me. You all know I wanted a little boy, a son to play for Man U, to piss Ben off with his Arsenal. I feel like I missed out—' she finished, her voice fading. A short silence followed Claire's confession.

'Group hug, group hug,' Ariel said quickly, throwing her arms wide to her friends, and Ben could hear, more than he could see, their movements towards each other. Just the way Claire sounded made him feel that if by a miracle, a hole could appear in the living room floor, he would gladly jump in.

That night after the Moon party was over and her friends gone, the worse for alcohol Claire went to bed in floods of tears. For a long while she was inconsolable. Ben held her in his arms as she cried.

'I'm sorry to be crying so often,' she said through sobs, 'I don't know what's wrong with me and I know it's no fucking fun for you.'

His heart softened at her despair and he pulled her in close, stroking her back and placing a kiss on her forehead. 'You've not long gone through an op, and you're probably crying because of the mistake you made.'

She moved her head to look at him. 'Mistake?'

'Yes. Saying any son we had would play for that team—I won't even mention their name and I'll thank you for not mentioning them in this house again.'

She laughed through her tears. 'I knew that would get you if you were listening. You've got poor Kenya in Arsenal kit; I figure our son could support Man U like his mother.'

'Would you really do that? Put a son of mine in that– that kit?'

'That's one dilemma we won't have,' she said sadly. 'Unless we go down the IVF route. I did some reading up on it, from the internet. The process seems tedious and the things my poor body would have to go through… all those hormones, and no guarantees.'

His stroking progressed from her back to under her vest top, cupping her breast, tweaking her nipples until her whimpering became desire-fuelled.

'You feel so good,' he whispered, his tongue circling her ear, ebbing towards her lips. He felt her mouth on his, hungry and urgent, opening so his tongue could explore.

'Oh, Benny… Benny, I just want us to be enough.'

He eased himself into her, feeling her moist warmth. 'You're enough for me.'

And in that moment he truly meant it.

Twenty
Kat
Jamaica

It was hard to wipe the smile off her face. Four passion-packed nights and five love-filled days with Ben had given her the high of a new bride. She felt Miss Ruthie's displeasure which was as blatant as that of a betrayed lover, her eyes silent with accusations and her lips resistant to words. Yet Kat could not pretend to be apologetic. She was not sorry for spending time in the arms of love, of the feeling of happiness that made her heart race or the desire that kept her moist. She wanted him. Not just his baby. She wanted all of him.

Rosie's words had disturbed her and for the first time she started thinking seriously about Claire-Louise. She hoped that Ben's wife could not compare to her. She somehow doubted this. Ben would demand love, passion and sweet, sweet sex from his woman. Jealousy was becoming a frequent visitor.

Columbus was more vocal. He had expressed outrage, arms flying around his head at her disappearing for so many days and not responding to her phone. Kat almost laughed at his theatrical displeasure and would have done so if he hadn't looked so forlorn and orphaned.

'Col, I really wish you and Miss Ruthie would stop this behaviour, it's not right,' she told him as they sat sipping ice lemonade on the veranda.

'It is not right that you should up and disappear for so many days without anyone knowing about your whereabouts or your safety. It was a selfish act, Kat.'

'How selfish? I left a note for Miss Ruthie, and I told her to let you know.'

'But we had no idea where you were! You're not long out of hospital, Dr Mattie said you should take it easy, yet you were off and we did not know where! Miss Ruthie was filled with worry.'

Kat took that on board. She could see the trauma Miss Ruthie would have suffered and that really wasn't her intention. But she wanted independence; she was going to be a mother herself and no longer wanted the fuss of a mother hen at her every turn.

'Miss Ruthie must learn to let me live my own life.' *And so must you*, she thought but left that unvoiced. Columbus was a sensitive soul and such a statement at such a time, she knew would crush him. His eyes questioned her, begged her for an answer as to where she had disappeared to. But she knew he was too proud to ask, that's why he had disguised it in Miss Ruthie's concern.

Her mobile rang and she answered it. 'Sweet girl.' Her heart sighed at the familiar voice. He rang every day, yet for every call her reaction was the same. Love made her want to leap. 'I waited for your call that didn't come last night; didn't you get my message?' Ben enquired. 'You need to call me every day because I worry you may leave me to pursue some other universe... seriously though, I worry.'

'Don't do that.' She smiled into the phone, fully aware that Columbus was turning an infuriating pink before her.

'Only one way to stop it,' he told her, 'let me have you, forever.'

'How would that work?'

'I'll find a way.'

'Do that, then ask me again.'

He laughed. 'You're sharp. You're miserable without me, aren't you?' he pleaded.

'Of course.'

'You don't sound miserable. Where are you? In bed?'

'No, it's early evening; I'm on the veranda with Columbus.'

'Why?'

She glanced at Columbus who was still keeping up his armour of disapproval, turning away from her and trying to look disinterested in her telephone conversation.

'That's a strange question,' she answered cautiously.

'No, it's not! Why is he hanging around you? You sure you told him about me? About us?'

Standing up, she walked down the steps and stood by the front gate, under the shade of the huge almond tree. She didn't want to have to answer Ben's questions with Columbus sitting there looking totally dejected.

'He knows about you, he's one of my best friends, Ben, don't make him a problem. Be more concerned about your own predicament.'

'For someone so calm you sure carry a mighty sting, Miss Lewis—but you can sting me any time... any place...

anywhere,' he lowered his voice suggestively.

She laughed. 'What shall I do with you? What will become of us, Ben?'

'Let's not go down your route of thoughts that takes us out of this universe.'

'One day we will have to, we have karma to face,' her voice carried a warning.

'One day doesn't have to be now... Love you, I'll call you tomorrow and don't forget to be miserable without me.'

She resumed her seat on the veranda and placing the phone on the table, she wearily looked at Columbus. His face wore a scowl and his eyes swam with pain. This was becoming increasingly uncomfortable for her. Columbus was a good friend and she did not want to hurt him.

'This is hard for you, Col, but you must understand. I'm happy now, more than I ever thought.'

'*Oui...* Yes,' he forced a pinched smile, '*Je vois...* I can see that.'

She felt the first flutter of her unborn at twenty-two weeks of pregnancy. Flutters so faint, like the flicker of butterfly wings. Her jeans and shorts were obviously too tight at last and looking down she could just about see her feet. It took everything she had not to tell Ben. The nearest she came to spilling her guts was to tell him about Mother Cynthy's dream of seeing her swimming with fishes and her nightmare about the suffocating fishes. He had laughed dubiously at her explanation of the meaning. She should have told him then but she couldn't. The fear of the unknown still loomed.

Twenty-one
Ben
London

Christmas was approaching and as the excitement of the festive season spread throughout his household, Ben could think only of Jamaica and Kat. The eight-foot organic tree with its silver, gold, green and red bulbs decorated by his daughters took centre stage in the living room. Claire had organised the shopping list via the internet, and the turkey, which Auntie Joan would prepare, was ordered from her friend's free range farm in Cornwall. Ben always left his own shopping to Auntie Joan. She bought everything; Claire's presents, the girls', the Professor's and his secretary's. The only gift he ever bought was Bubs'. This year he had Kat's to think about, which was proving a task, knowing her as he now did. She was so unfussy. He eventually decided to put some money in her bank account, that way she could choose her own gift.

He had spoken to Kat the previous night and she sounded faint, nothing to do with the distance. Was she ill? He had asked and she was quick to assure him that she was merely tired and recovering from the flu. It was three months since he last saw her and it was becoming increasingly unbearable, this distance of sea, sky and miles. The urge to have her at hand had reached fever pitch. He was trapped between two worlds, two women and an unrealistic plan of having them both.

When you walk into the office of Thornton Benjamin, you know you are in the presence of success. The office housed heavy mahogany furniture, thick carpet and expensive African and Asian artwork on the walls. The busy people, in and out, the telephone going constantly with investors wanting to invest in or buy properties abroad all rang success. He was dressed in a finely tailored dark blue Oswald Boateng suit, with a crisp sky blue and white striped shirt and a red silk tie. On his feet, his shoes were dark brown highest quality supple leather that looked as if they cost a small fortune. He stood gazing out the window of his seventeenth floor city office building. He could see the London Eye and many other iconic landmarks all united along the meandering banks of the River Thames. He would like to one day show Kat this sight at night, when the lights transformed it into wonderland. He felt sure she would whip out her pad and pencil and start sketching. The thought erupted a laugh. The next time he spoke to her he would offer her a holiday in London, book her into the Marriot in Park Lane and pretend he had out of London business to attend to. If he planned it right it could work, he felt both sure and guilty.

A feeling of melancholy plagued him. Maybe it was the Christmas Carols playing softly in the background or the happy giggles of the young PAs and secretaries who were enjoying the flirtatious atmosphere alcohol and Christmas brought. The combination was actually lethal. Too many broken marriages, relationships or lives happened because of an office Christmas affair, one-night stand or simply a drunken kiss. Or maybe it was not having Kat beside him to share Christmas with. He wondered what she would do for the holidays. If she would take her daily walk down to the beach to meditate on her throne of stone. Or go up to Meadow View to watch the speeding boats or even just sit by the river and ponder those trips on shooting stars and outer universes. There was so much to love about her and so much standing between them.

He sat at his desk and automatically picked up a pen and without thinking wrote her initials, *KL*. Then he sketched a heart shape around it and laughed at his childish moment. The phone on his desk purred.

'Yes, Carmen!' he said sharply. 'I have no appointments booked in and—'

'There are three people on their way in to see you... a surprise, they say.'

Before he could respond his office door flew open and Claire and the girls filled the space. He quickly scribbled over *KL* and felt a twinge in his chest. He had the urge to cry, erasing her like that.

'Daddy!' Kenya, dressed in her Arsenal kit under her fur coat rushed towards him, her arms wide.

The urge left him and he scooped up his daughter. She was a tomboy and at five years old still young enough not to care. India on the other hand was fast approaching eleven and could tell you which designer dressed which stars and was opposed to wearing anything that wasn't a name brand. He and Claire would have to work to alter that part of her.

'Come on, Daddy, we've come to drag you out to cheer you up. You've been too busy lately.' India tugged at his arm.

'Really? You noticed something other than your hair, nails and clothes?' he teased.

She hit him playfully.

'They certainly have.' Claire walked over and kissed him. 'You've ducked out of too many weekend activities,' she said meaningfully. He understood. Guilt entwined with affection made him pull her in, and cupping her face with both hands he kissed her, lingeringly, his eyes closed wondering what the hell he was going to do.

'Yuk, you guys, let's go and eat.' India pushed her parents teasingly.

'Daddy! That's you!' Kenya suddenly squealed. Ben looked at what his daughter was pointing; it was his sketch, the portrait Kat had completed which he had mounted on canvas and framed in mahogany to match his office furniture.

Claire turned to see what her daughter was so excited about. She walked closer to the drawing. 'Wow! That is remarkable.' She folded her arms and tilted her head to one side. 'The artist is good. He certainly captured something. Your hair needed doing, but you look stunning. Who's KL?' she asked, reading the signature at the bottom of the picture.

'Can I have it in my bedroom? It's brilliant!' India added. 'You look real handsome, like a movie star.'

'I'm totally impressed. Who's the artist?' Claire asked again.

'Why? You want one done too?' Ben teased, his heart in his mouth, his mind searching for some obscure name he could give her.

She laughed. 'No, couldn't sit long enough for that, give me a photo any day. But I think he caught a side of you that I've never seen. You look... different. Were you on a beach? The palm tree—'

'I got it done in Jamaica,' he said quickly. 'You get some real talent out there.'

Claire looked taken aback. 'Jamaica. Who—'

'Can we go now?' Kenya's impatience saved her father from any more explanations.

London is a magical hub nearing Christmas. The colourful flashing lights in the shops and the extravagant window displays of Santa or the nativity play lined the high streets. The market stalls were laden with colourful festive goods, tinsels, toys, games and the friendly good-natured proprietors made great festive efforts in their Santa hats and coats. The sweet, tantalising smells of cinnamon and vanilla, of baked bread, spiced buns and Christmas pudding wafted out from the bakery, filling noses and enticing taste buds. The lift in people's mood could be attributed to the joviality that paved the streets, the buses and the tubes. You can't get completely away from the drunken and obnoxious behaviour of a few individuals, but overall that too was tolerated, even if an undertone of disgust pursued.

They drove down to Hyde Park where Ben parked the car on a side road and they walked through the huge grounds, the girls running ahead of their entwined parents. He realised then that he had not seen a park in the Meadows, not in the form that existed in London, never walked in a park with Kat.

Claire smiled at her husband. 'Are you okay, Benny?'

'Course I am.'

'I know there's something on your mind, I know it. You go far away sometimes and I'm wondering if you're getting the seven-year itch at eleven years of marriage because I still love being married to you.'

'Well I do manage to keep you in your Prada and Gucci...'

She threw him a punch and he winced in mock pain.

'Anything worrying you, business going alright?'

'Am I in for an inquisition here?' He grimaced. 'Yes, business is great. Very busy as you see.'

'So nothing is worrying you?'

'No.'

'Do you still desire me...?'

'What a question. Yes. You know I do.'

'I know. But I like to hear it, you know, like you want me like no other. A woman likes to hear her man tell her those things more often. Sometimes you go some place in your mind that I can't,' she insisted.

'Then forgive me.' He didn't want to lie, to deny her her true feelings because they had been correct and he was feeling bad enough.

'So, my husband, what gift have you bought me this year?' She pressed against him.

'You wait and see,' he replied, enveloping her in his arms.

'In Jamaica, did you get tempted by some hot Jamaican booty?' She was joking of course, but Ben froze.

She was still in his arms so she didn't see the look on his face. She thought his stiffened structure was a tease and hugged him even more, laughing.

He recovered quickly. 'Yes. Plenty. I was spoilt for choice every night.'

He felt lucky she laughed and released him. 'Mummy was asking why we're not having Christmas dinner by them this year?'

'Oh Claire, tell her because we did last year, and every year since we've been married. This year we'll stay home and she and Albert are welcome to join us, but I want a Christmas at home this year. Every year one of us has to be sober for the drive home—in our own home we can both get stoned out of our head and hit the bed, get creative until the early hours.'

She burst into fits of laughter. 'Oh Benny, when you're drunk, you can't even find your dick to piss.'

He joined in her laughter but it was hard to relax, to let go and get some of that Christmas spirit when everything lacked certainty and guilt wouldn't exit his thoughts.

Twenty-two
Miss Ruthie

Kat moved lethargically, Miss Ruthie noted as she watched her dressing for church the Sunday morning ten days before Christmas. Her heart housed fear at her daughter's predicament because of her sister-in-law Doris. Her only hope was her prayers to Sweet Jesus and Mother Cynthy, who had assured her of Kat's survival.

'Kat, you not looking good, you feeling alright?' Miss Ruthie's concern caused her to lose the frosty formality that had persisted since discovering Kat's pregnancy.

'Sorry to cause you so much worry, Miss Ruthie. I really didn't want to make your spirit so vex.' Kat sounded breathless.

'Neva mind that, how you sounding so tired. You betta not come with me to church today. Stay home, rest little bit.'

'I think you're right, I do feel...' Kat swallowed with difficulty, reaching for something to lean on. 'I think I should go to the hospital.'

Miss Ruthie froze as she looked at Kat and then she rushed onto the veranda and down the stairs with the swiftness of a prey under attack. She shouted to Tin-Tin, her neighbour's son to hurry and fetch Columbus and Old Man. They would need Columbus' jeep and she would need Old Man's calm confidence in everything turning out alright. But Tin-Tin's mother called back to say he had gone to the river. Miss Ruthie returned to her house in even more of a panic to find Kat curled in the foetal position on her bed, rocking to and fro. She was sweating profusely, her breathing shallow. Miss Ruthie rushed to her.

'Kat, Kat...' She wiped her child's brow. 'You havin' a crisis but Tin-Tin isn't home, I'll run to de post office and use de phone to fetch Columbus and Old Man.'

Kat gave a small pain filled smile. 'I phoned Columbus on my mobile, he'll be here soon... with Old Man... don't you fret... it's not a crisis, my water's broken. I can handle this, Miss Ruthie, my contractions are nothing compared to—'

'Oh, Sweet Jesus! It's far too soon.' Miss Ruthie's panic-filled voice dislodged Kat's calm demeanour.

Kat clutched her mother's hand fearfully. 'Don't let nothing happen to my baby, please, Miss Ruthie, please, please.'

'You feeling plenty pain? Oh Kat, why you so stubborn? Why do this to yourself?' she cried alarmingly. Then she placed a hand on Kat's damp forehead and started praying. 'Oh, Sweet Jesus, help her, help her please, watch over my child! You delivered her to me, and I know you have the power to take her back! Oh gentle Sweet Jesus, so meek and mild, look upon my little child and suffer her to live another day... Amen... Amen in Jesus' name!'

Miss Ruthie had not missed a day of her regular Sunday worship since she had given birth to Kat all those years ago. Ever since then she had taken her regular seat in the front row of Holy Mother of God Church. Today everyone would see she wasn't there and no doubt Nellie Potato would create speculation. Since discovering Kat's condition, the inquisitive Nellie Potato had taken to dropping by more than her customary morning visits, her eyes scanning Kat for evidence of the rumours she had heard. Miss Ruthie remained tight-lipped and defensive, making it quite obvious that she was not going to discuss anything about Kat, much to Nellie Potato's disappointment.

The riotous winds carried the white sheet of rain and lashed it against the windows of the hospital while raucous thunder roared across the bleached-out sky. Christmas wasn't a rainy time of year in the Meadows and Miss Ruthie was forced to think about what Old Man said about global warming. She couldn't quite bring herself to believe in it though, as far as she was concerned God was responsible for controlling the weather, not some scientific explanation of mankind's waste. God was responsible for all things, including Kat's life.

The tall gowned figure of Doctor Mattie came towards her and she reached for Old Man's hand, gripping him in panic and expecting the worse. *Kat didn't make it*, her mind screamed. *That wretched parasite has eaten away at my child and has swallowed her life!*

The cry was harsh, unrecognisable as it struggled from the confines of her throat. She heard herself but could do nothing to stop it. She became aware of Old Man's arms tightening around her shoulders but she couldn't stop the sound forcing its way out of her mouth.

'No... no... no... nooooooooooooo!'

'Please, Miss Ruthie, please sit down and stop that screaming, Kat is alright, she's okay... and the baby too. It's a little boy, he's fine, small but strong. We'll keep an eye on him in Special Care for a month, but he's fine.' Dr Mattie's voice was firm and sympathetic at the same time. 'Kat's going to be alright.' The doctor smiled brightly.

Columbus sighed, releasing air loudly. 'She's going to be fine, Miss Ruthie, she made it... she made it!'

Old Man Jaguar circled her with his arms and she fell against him, glad for the strength of his chest and the faint smell of lavender and baby powder on his clothing. She sobbed into his shirt, whispering a prayer. 'Oh God, Oh God, Oh God... Thank you, Sweet Jesus, thank you.'

Kat was still sleeping from the anaesthetic when Miss Ruthie entered her room. Her hair was coal black, sprawled out on the whiteness of the pillow. She had a drip in her left hand but no other tubes. A smile rested on her lips and she looked as though her dreams were enjoyable and private.

'If your daddy could only see you now!' Miss Ruthie spoke softly. She opened her hand bag, took out a comb and began running it through Kat's hair. It had been many years since she had combed her child's hair. Then she had her firmly between her thighs and meted out the occasional conk to her head when Kat had fidgeted. She placed her bag on the chair so that she could get to grips with her hair. It had grown, but then pregnancy was a time when hair had a good growth spurt.

'You going to be alright,' she spoke softly as she started to part and plait Kat's hair.

She plaited it in two, just like when she was a child. 'I mad like hell with you, girl! You had to put yourself through this... and for what! That little parasite nearly take you from me. Don't do this again, you hearing me? Don't you ever!'

Dr Mattie told her Kat would be sleeping for a few more hours and insisted that she went to see her grandson. Miss Ruthie was adamant that she did not want to see him. He had caused so much trouble and wasn't even an hour old. Dr Mattie would not give up and eventually Miss Ruthie gave in, taking Old Man with her.

She was not prepared for the tide of emotions that engulfed her as she saw her tiny grandson for the first time.

'Look, Old Man,' she whispered, amazed, 'look at how un-creased he is.' Tears unexpectantly filled her eyes. Kat had a baby, her daughter had a baby.

Old Man gently squeezed her shoulders as they marvelled at the baby's light brown skin and mop of copper soft curls.

'He looks like his father,' Old Man pointed out. 'The button nose is Kat's and Glenrick's before her, but his lips and forehead, that's his daddy's.'

Miss Ruthie was disappointed that he didn't house her heritage. It would have been nice if she could see something of herself in him. The baby suddenly yawned, his little fists cupped his cheeks and a shadow of a smile played around his tiny mouth. His eyes momentarily fluttered open, taking even more of her heart.

'It's early days yet,' Old Man said, 'but I think he has Kat's smile and Kat's smile belongs to her mother.'

The warmth she felt for her grandson surprised Miss Ruthie. She repented too, for wishing such ills on a poor unborn and promised herself that she would fast for three days to wipe out the stain of the sin. She felt she should be happier but something about the whole event—Kat becoming pregnant, Kat keeping it a secret from the foreigner, Kat changing so much—the whole thing sat like a lump of rock in her chest and it didn't seem to be going anywhere too fast.

Twenty-three

Kat

The first moment Kat was able to hold her son, she fell in love. She had never seen anyone so small and so perfect, and she marvelled at the fact that he came from her. She had done what everyone thought she would never do and she now had what the town thought she never would. Her own baby. His soft baby curls came low on his forehead and ran in a straight line down the sides of his face, ending by his ear lobes. When he opened his eyes, they were his father's, hazel green and round. His nose was snub and his lips a full pout.

On her first day home from the hospital with the baby, Miss Ruthie had shut down the shop for the day and got Columbus to write a sign saying *No Visitors*. She wanted to keep the gossips, particularly Nellie Potato in suspense.

'The first thing we must do is get him an age paper from the registry. What name you want?' Miss Ruthie spoke with an edge to her voice. Kat knew her mother's anger was still ripe despite the adoration she looked at her grandson with. Miss Ruthie would eventually want an apology and an explanation.

'Shadrach Thornton Benjamin Lewis,' Kat announced proudly.

'So that's his father's name.' Columbus was solemn even as his little finger was held in a grip by the baby.

Kat did not respond. She held a miracle in her arms and she wanted to etch this feeling in a place that she could revisit often.

'Don't you think you should let the father know now?' Ruthie pointed out sternly.

Again Kat did not respond. She may have to explain about Ben later but for now, this was her moment with her son.

Life was changed forever. Now there were three of them in the small house. Kat was pleasantly surprised by the changes Columbus made to her bedroom to accommodate a small cradle and chest of drawers. The ceiling and the walls had been painted baby blue and new curtains and bed linen had transformed the look. It had been a month since she slept in her own bed and here she was at home with her own baby.

She waited for Miss Ruthie to leave the room before reaching for her mobile phone. It had been switched off and she knew Ben would be frantic. She was apprehensive, no ideas forming as to what she would say about her silence.

'Kat! Kat, what's going on? Where have you been? Are you okay? I've been calling you and I'm out of my mind with worry, what's going on?' Ben's words tumbled out with the gush of a confused and upset child. 'I didn't know what to think, I didn't know if anything had happened to you, my God, what is going on with you?

Don't you know I worry, really worry when I can't get hold of you?'

Tears sprung to her eyes. 'Yes.'

'What happened? Are you okay? You sound tired. Have you been ill?'

She seized that opportunity. 'Yes.'

'It doesn't mean you can't use a phone. What's really going on, Kat? Something is. I called to wish you Merry Christmas... no connection. I called to wish you happy New Year... no connection. Nothing! For so long! I mean, talk to me, what is going on?'

It wasn't going to be as easy as she thought. Her silence brought irritation to his voice.

'You have someone else? You want out? Be honest with me, don't play me now! Is it this so called best friend, the French guy?'

'No! Col is my friend, how many times will I have to tell you? There's no-one else. I'm sorry, I should have called but sometimes everyday life and events get in the way and my life is very different from yours... It's not a justifiable reason, but it's my reason. I'm sorry to have worried you, Ben.'

His voice softened. 'I do worry about you, Kat. Despite all we share, all we mean to each other, there's a part of you that I can't reach. It's like you deliberately lock that part of you away. Is it because of the situation?' They never spoke about Claire-Louise or his marriage; it was always referred to as 'the situation.'

'I guess so.' She was part telling the truth. Shadrach had brought new feelings, a new reality to be faced.

'We have to talk. I'm coming out to the Meadows for Easter. It's three months away and it feels like years, but

I'll be able to stay for a month. In the meantime, will you please answer my calls?'

'Yes, Ben. I'll be here.'

'I put some money into your account for Christmas, and I really don't want to hear from your independence right now.'

She wasn't going to object. She would need all the financial help she could get.

'Thank you, Ben, it's so considerate of you.'

'Are you miserable without me?'

She laughed. 'Of course.'

The journey home had been exhausting and the call to Ben exhilarating. She had three months to prepare herself for what would be a revelation for Ben. Fear hovered around. The fear that perhaps he would see it as deceit and her a liar. The tables had now turned and she was the one with the secret. Yes, fear was powerful, but the hope that he would be happy beyond belief won over.

Once her baby was asleep in his cradle, she buried herself beneath the sheets and inhaled, whispering as sleep seeped in like the waves on the shores, 'Ben, you have a son... we have a son.'

On Shadrach's six week check and her own post-natal, Kat was given the all clear and her immediate thought was to go down to the beach and dig her fingers and toes into the sand. But Columbus looked as horrified as Miss Ruthie when she mentioned her intention and so she settled herself on the veranda with him fussing over her. Miss Ruthie had taken Shadrach to visit Pastor

Tuff and his wife and Kat knew her mother would be discussing christening arrangements.

'*Shaddy est un très beau bébé...* Shaddy is a good-looking little baby.' Columbus adjusted a cushion behind her back. 'Looks like his daddy, I take it.' His tone begged answers.

'I should explain a few things to you, Col.' She waited for him to pull the chair closer. 'You will never understand what I did, but I did it and I don't regret it.'

'Why him?' It had been the predominant question burning in Columbus' head ever since she announced her planned pregnancy.

'I told you on my sixteenth birthday Mother Cynthy told me that a man from across the sea would give me a baby. At first I thought it was you,' she laughed. 'I didn't plan meeting him, Col, but when I did... I wanted to have his child more than anything... It was predicted. It's my fate.'

Columbus looked frustrated with her answer.

'What I'm about to tell you now must be held secret under our bond of friendship.'

Columbus nodded.

'Ben is married, Columbus. He has two daughters.'

'What?'

'You heard me correct. Don't look at me like that. I didn't know at first and when I found out, I loved him too much to walk away.'

'What?'

She shifted in the chair and repeated, 'You heard me correct. I love him.'

'You are crazy, no? You are very crazy, in here.' He pointed to his head.

She nodded. 'I know. I was angry with him for lying at first, but by then, it was too late,' she hugged herself and sniffed back her tears. 'He was already in my soul, Col.'

'What future do you see?'

Kat eased herself out of the chair and put distance between herself and Columbus by standing on the second step of the stairs. She looked up to the sky, still holding herself. 'I don't know.'

Columbus heaved frustration. 'And when he finds out about his son... *et puis quoi?* What then?'

'He'll accept Shaddy. I'll explain things. It will be much better face to face, and when he actually sees Shaddy, he won't stay mad for long, he just won't. He'll want his son.'

His look told her he could not even begin to comprehend what she had done, and she couldn't confess that deep, deep down she had reservations. Ben had a life. He loved his wife and his children. Where exactly did she fit into this?

'You think it will be that easy? You tricked a guy into getting you pregnant—'

'I didn't trick Ben. I hoped to get pregnant but I didn't know if I would... That was an act of God, not a trick.'

'Now you sound like Miss Ruthie. What world do you live in? If you knowingly get pregnant for a married man without his knowledge or consent, that is called a trick. I don't think you realise the implications. I'm quite certain this guy wouldn't have told his wife about his fling.'

'I didn't know he was married when we first had sex,

and we didn't have a fling,' Kat scolded. 'We have love. He calls me every day and if he doesn't hear from me, he worries. It's real what we have... but it is complicated, Mother Cynthy said it would be.'

'Kat, *ma chérie, écoute*... you sound like a teenager in denial. I'm trying to make you see sense. If he hasn't told his wife about you, then it will be a shock to her and he may not thank you for giving him a child he never asked for.'

Columbus slowly joined her on the stairs, facing her full on. 'From where I'm standing I think you need to rethink. I do believe that you are clear in your intentions, but they are not right. I still can't believe you planned the whole thing. *Dis-moi*, tell me, did you try it with anyone else? How many more potential fathers did you try before getting lucky?'

She ignored him with a shoulder shrug because she understood the root of his sarcasm was his personal pain and because answering questions which had no merit was never her priority.

'God forbid, but if anything should ever happen to me and I can't look after Shaddy, I have one wish: please phone Ben and tell him about his son. That's all you have to do. And you must do it for me, Col, have I ever asked you for anything before?'

She watched the fight leave him like water down a plug hole. Over the years of friendship she had asked for nothing and accepted very little.

'Alright,' he breathed in resignation. 'Kat, *ma chérie*... I'll do it, even though you ask too much.'

'I know.' Her heart ached at the anguish on his face and she wished for one moment she could love him the way he wanted. 'I'm sorry, Col, it seems I've given you a sponge to dry up the sea.'

Twenty-four

Ben

London

London looked like a postcard out of a Christmas collection with the snow resting on rooftops, trees, bushes and cars. It was February and the snow had come far too late for Christmas. It had been his worst Christmas and New Year because he had been unable to reach Kat by phone. During the long month of not hearing her voice, he had once again considered doing the crazy thing of jumping on a plane and walking to her doorstep. He was stopped only by common sense. Her explanation had infuriated him, as he couldn't help feeling that perhaps she had got involved with someone else, maybe that best friend of hers; the Frenchman Columbus. On eventually hearing her voice softened by warmth, desire and love, he was able to push that thought out of his head. Her love was always convincing and he was very happy that she still wanted him.

He had a surprise for her and hoped it would be a welcomed surprise, one that would not cause her strenuous objections, as was her custom when given gifts. He had to prove to her that he was serious about their relationship, despite the situation, and felt the move he had made would confirm his love for her. The solicitors had informed him that all the deeds for the property would be completed long before Easter. It was a three-bedroom town house in the leafy suburbs of Meadow View, with a front and back garden, and a veranda overlooking the sea in the distance. Surely her mother, the notorious Miss Ruthie would not pass up the opportunity to live in such a prestigious area and in such a wonderful house. And Kat. Would this not prove to her that she was in his long-term plan?

Ben looked at his watch. Midday, meaning it would be 6am in Jamaica. Briefly looking at the door he picked up the phone and called her.

'Hello?'

'I love it when your voice sounds all coated in sleep, it reminds me of our nights between the sheets.'

'Ben.'

'My sweet girl.' He could hear her breath. 'I've been thinking about you... Let me buy you a home, Kat, so when I come we have our own place.'

Her silence was loud.

'We're more than hotel rooms, Kat.'

'So you want to buy me a house to live in on my own and wait around for when you can come and spend some time with me? Is this what you're offering?' she responded hotly.

'I'm trying, Kat.'

'What exactly are you trying?'

He sighed into the phone. 'I'm trying my best to keep you. I don't want to lose you.'

The door to his study burst open. 'Daddy, Daddy!'

Kenya stood holding her favourite Pooh Bear by the ear, tears threatening to erupt.

'I'll call you back,' Ben quickly clicked the phone off but not before hearing her rather dry sarcastic laugh.

'I'm too big for this Pooh Bear, I want to give him to Mummy's charity and India says I can't.' Her voice wobbled with tears.

'I told her it's torn and old, I would feel insulted if someone gave me something like that.' India suddenly appeared behind her, hand on hip in that authoritative way she had over her younger sister.

'But you said we mustn't waste anything,' she spoke accusingly to her father.

'But Mummy told me to make sure the donations are decent,' India retorted.

'My Pooh Bear is decent.'

'Isn't.'

'Is.'

'Isn't.'

'Oh come on girls, stop arguing. India, don't tease your little sister about a toy bear.'

He beckoned to Kenya and she ran into his arms.

'Listen, baby girl. I think you have a wonderful kind heart, but Pooh is a little battered,' he spoke softly, stroking her hair.

'Told you,' India piped.

Her words caused Kenya to burst into uncontrollable sobs, and she buried her face into her father's neck.

'India!' Ben spoke firmly. 'Go and find something useful to do before I find it for you.'

India scuttled away, mumbling that she was only telling the truth.

'It's okay, baby, it's okay.' He soothed Kenya, stroking her back until her sobs became little sniffles. 'I'm going down to the Professor's, you want to come with me?'

'Yes,' she sniffed.

'Go ask Auntie Joan to put some clothes on you.'

Kenya ran out calling out for Auntie Joan and bumped into her mother. 'Sorry, Mummy, I'm going to the Professor's with Daddy.'

'Make sure you wrap up warm, you had that chesty cough last week.'

Claire walked towards her husband, clad from head to toe in a long cream suede coat with white fur collar and matching Russian fur hat, and on her feet, flat, white Gestapo-looking leather boots.

'I'm going now.' Claire bent to kiss his lips. 'Got my Lupus meeting then having lunch with Helen. This week has been hell getting the end of year accounts ready, I need a break.'

'How about taking India along, she'd benefit from spending some more time with you.'

'Can you take her with you? She gets bored with my meetings.'

'I know. But I think she might benefit from spending more time with you.' He added quickly, 'She's becoming quite a little madam and I think it's an attention-seeking thing. She keeps teasing Kenya.'

'Oh that's a sibling thing. I teased my sister all the time. And anyway, Kenya can be too sensitive sometimes, a bit like you.' She pinched his nose, leading him to smile.

'And just remember India is all hormones right now, whether you accept it or not... Benny, are you listening? You do that so often lately—daydreaming.'

His smile came from far away. Kat lived in his mind. Where else could he go to find her apart from the memories wrapped within his thoughts?

'I guess I've been overdoing things—'

'Yes, you have. The planning for the annual Lupus ball is coming on really well, you can read my speech later.' She didn't wait for a response; she wrapped her arms around his neck and kissed him lightly. 'I might be late, but wait up.'

He watched the closed door for a long time, the taste of her kiss still in his mouth and the mist from her perfume filling his nose. He closed his eyes and saw them both. Claire and Kat.

The situation had gotten out of his control and something had to give. He felt strongly about abandonment and rejection. He knew first-hand the damage and the poison it left, dear God, he didn't want to be associated with such acts.

Twenty-five
Kat

Kat stood naked in front of her full-length mirror, viewing herself critically. She had been disappointed to have escaped stretch marks and still maintain her slender form. Her only consolation was the fading scar from the caesarean and her breasts, despite ceasing the feeding of her baby, remained a size bigger. It was not her decision to halt the breast feeding, but Miss Ruthie at every opportunity pointed out how the weight was melting off her already meagre body.

'You're being sucked dry!' she accused. Kat had felt pressured into cutting that intimate bond with her baby, but eventually accepted the idea because of the implication of breast milk leaking all over Ben during their love making.

As Easter beckoned and Ben's arrival neared, she began to feel fearful. The possibility that she had so far refused to consider lost its transparency and appeared within reach before her. Ben could actually be furious with her, or consider what she did a deception. He could, as Columbus said, feel betrayed and disappointed.

Her baby's cooing filled the room. She dressed and

picked him up, kissing his plump cheeks. He smiled and she laughed, all fears disintegrating like ice in the sun. Surely Ben would love this bundle of joy; his son looked so much like him.

'Kat,' Miss Ruthie interrupted her flow of thoughts as she entered the room. 'Pastor Tuff set the date for Shaddy's blessing. Easter Morning. The contractors will finish the building work before then, we can have the party on the front lawn. Of course Mother Cynthy will be one of the Godmothers.'

Miss Ruthie had waited nigh on thirty years for her indoor kitchen and bathroom to be installed. Columbus and Old Man were overseeing the contractors.

'Yes,' she agreed. Her brain leaped into search mode as she sought ways to postpone the event. Ben was due to arrive that very afternoon. It wouldn't be a good time for him to discover the existence of his son.

'Why so soon?' Her casual tone belied the turmoil she felt inside. 'Easter is only a month away.'

'Plenty time to get things ready. You might like to make Old man a Godfather as well as Columbus. They both been helpful to us.'

Kat felt panicked. It would mean catastrophe if Ben turned up at Shadrach's christening before being told about him.

'I also think you should phone the father, he must contribute to Shaddy's upbringing. It not right you not telling him. How we going to manage the whole christening party? Everyone will expect to eat and drink. We must invite folks or they will talk.'

'I don't care,' Kat blurted out. 'You never even asked me about my own baby's blessing. Suppose I have other plans for that day? Did you even consider that?'

Miss Ruthie stared in open-mouthed alarm at her daughter's outburst. Kat did not care at this point, all she knew was that she was not ready to reveal all to Ben; it had to be done in her time. It was so typical of Miss Ruthie to take control and barge ahead like a tank without brakes. At first she had been distant and acted like she wanted nothing to do with her grandson, then as the weeks progressed, she became more active and vocal about the way she believed her grandson should be reared. Now she had just gone ahead with plans without consulting her. Kat was furious. But mostly anxious.

'And what plans? You never tell me 'bout no plans! Not that you tell me anything. What plan is more important than a child's blessing?'

Tears welled in Kat's eyes but she blinked them back. She could not tell Miss Ruthie about Ben's visit. Perhaps she could attend the Christening then sneak away to see him. But for how long could she keep this up? Her nerves were a wreck as the time drew near for Ben to come. She rehearsed a thousand times the words she would use to tell him about his son. Now she wished she had done it sooner, why hadn't she told him when she found out she was pregnant, why? She felt hopeless, like her world had been given a shaking and everything was now floating, unsettled in chaos around her.

The indoor kitchen and bathroom were completed a week before the Christening. Miss Ruthie had been saving nigh on thirty years for this. It was the first time Kat had seen her stay happy for so long. She sang whenever she took a shower, in fact she spent most of her time in the kitchen singing or humming. In the meantime Kat was becoming more anxious.

The evening before Ben was due to arrive, he phoned while Miss Ruthie organised Old Man to tidy the yard and set out chairs.

His familiar voice greeted her, but sounded unusually flat. 'Sweet girl, how's it going?'

'Is anything wrong? Are you sick?'

'No, not sick, well not physically, but I'm as mad as hell.'

'Why?'

'My trip for tomorrow, cancelled. The company out there has signed a contract with an American company at the last minute so they've cancelled my trip.'

Kat didn't know whether to laugh or cry. She of course wanted to see him, longed for him, his kisses and the feel of his arms, but this gave her more time to prepare him for his son and to prepare herself for his reaction. God doesn't give you what you can't bear, was one of Miss Ruthie's many mantras, and Miss Ruthie was right. God had seen that Ben's coming now, at the same time as Shadrach's blessing would have been a catastrophe.

'That's too bad, Ben, I was looking forward to seeing you... to spend days and nights,' she replied truthfully.

'You sure? You don't sound too upset. I thought I was in for a long lecture on keeping promises. You missing me? Make sure you're miserable without me you know.'

She laughed. 'You're such a doubter. If you don't know how much I love you by now, when will you?'

'When I can have you near me all the time?'

She looked at the phone and wondered how possible this really was.

Twenty-six

Ben

London

Ben was finding it difficult to act normal that Easter. All his hopes had been set on going to Jamaica, to the Meadows and to Kat. How cruel fate was, to bring him so close to seeing her again, then to snatch it away like a big tease. He fought to hide the misery that cantered within.

'What? You haven't had the time to read my speech but you daydream all the time?'

Claire stood sulkily before him, her arms folded. The whole family had come for a day out at the Southbank to a reading by India's favourite author, Malorie Blackman. The Professor had taken the girls into the hall and Claire had stopped Ben from going in. Her eyes were pleading and Ben knew he lived too many hours alone in his head.

'I'll read it as soon as we get home, I swear,' he said, holding a hand on his heart.

'Are you having an affair, Benny?' Claire, her eyes narrowed by suspicion and her mouth made sulky by mood, confronted him. 'I have no evidence; when you're not working you're either home, out with Bubs, colleagues or the Professor. But what is it I feel?'

Ben was too scared to attempt an explanation at this stage. It would make matters worse, he was sure. He wasn't brave enough or ready to disrupt his daughters' lives and admit that he loved another woman. He also loved his wife and did not want to leave her, destroy what they had.

He hoped his smile was dismissive. 'Now what would make you say a thing like that? It's all in your head.' He wished he could find the sincerity in the words he spoke and didn't need to look at her to know she remained unconvinced. The confusion that had settled within him was maddening. Despite every conversation with Kat and every moment with her wrapped in his arms after passion spent, he still loved Claire. *How absurd*, he chastised himself. Maybe it would be easier if he loved one more than the other, but he didn't.

'I asked you before if we were okay and I have to ask it again because you're changed... something's going on with you,' she said sadly. 'You don't seem too bothered about making love to me so much, so who is she?'

Ben knew he had been naive to think she would not notice his shift. He thought her busy social life would have kept her absorbed. He had misjudged her.

'What are you talking about? Sweet girl, of course I love making love with you, but for a while you were off me, remember?'

'Yes,' she admitted ruefully, 'so are you trying to make me suffer for that?' She pouted.

Guilt engulfed him. 'Let's get away for Easter,' he suggested and watched as hope and relief replaced the frustration and suspicion in her eyes. 'Just you and me.'

It was an act of spontaneity and desperation.

'Where?'

'Jamaica.' The word was out before he could stem the highly dangerous thought. Even now as he was trying to avoid causing his wife any further turbulence, he was also mapping out a way to see his mistress.

Claire hissed displeasure. 'Haven't you had enough of that place? It's really made an impression on you.'

Ben changed the destination swiftly. 'Okay, let's go to Italy or Spain, they have great beaches... or even Florida, you choose.'

He wasn't going to push Jamaica. His head was already taking control knowing the kind of trouble his heart could get him into. Jamaica was an irrational idea, he conceded.

Claire didn't have to think long. 'Italy sounds good.'

Twenty-seven
Kat
Jamaica

Easter arrived with rumbling dark moving clouds. A turbulent summer ahead, the town folks forecasted. Shadrach's blessing was going according to Miss Ruthie's plan with most of the Christian town attending. Blessings, weddings and funerals always turned Christian folk out in their best dress, and it was expected and accepted that they should turn up whether they were invited or not, whether they were known to you or not. Kat was not happy about this and wanted it scaled down to the few people she knew with genuine hearts, but Miss Ruthie's will of steel had matched her own. And with Ben no longer coming, a great pillar of burden had been removed from her mind.

'It's the way things are done! At your blessing the whole town came with gifts, good will and prayers. Be grateful, child.'

'They come with bad minds too. All they want is to see who my baby looks like. They can't believe that me, Katherine Lewis, the girl full of sickness has a baby. They want to come and see if he has the sickness too. Some are saying that Col is the father, others are saying it's some drug-pushing foreigner—I don't want those hypocrites near my baby.'

'Your mouth too harsh, Kat. It's the way things are done and who are you to want to change it!'

Kat did manage to stand her ground in having Rosie as a Godmother, and Paula, even though she wouldn't make it to Jamaica. Rosie came with Ras Solomon and her five children, washed, dressed in worn but clean clothes and behaving impeccably.

There were two parts to a Blessing. First, Shadrach's christening by Pastor Harper where the choir, dressed in purple and white sang in harmonious tones to the sound of the organ and their own clapping hands. Then there was the second half back at the house where Mother Cynthy wrapped a blue cloth around the baby and walked him one hundred yards away from the crowd to whisper a name in his ear. This name she revealed only to his mother and it would only be used in times of trouble. Should the child depart from the good ways of the Lord, then the mother would have to gather all the Godparents present at the time of his Blessing and they would circle him while she sang his name in his ear. This would remind him of the time when he was pure and no sin could enter his soul, which would bring him back to who he was.

Once the ceremony was over people began eating, drinking and enjoying the sound of their own voices. They congratulated Kat on her 'pretty' son, satisfied themselves that the child looked healthy and that indeed was not Columbus' son as was suspected, but that of a foreigner. She had never missed Ben as much as she did now, alone at the blessing of their son and Ben not having an inkling of the baby's existence. The tears were close. She didn't know it would be this hard. She thought having her baby would fill all her lonely moments, fulfil all her dreams, she knew now that he only increased them. Ben. She needed him.

Kat handed Shadrach to Rosie and made her escape from the rowdy crowd. She walked far enough down the lane for their noise to become a distant hum before taking out her mobile phone.

'Ben... Ben,' she said when he answered her call.

'Hey, sweet girl.'

'I miss you. I wish... I just wish.' Passion filled her tone and she wanted to confess everything to him.

His laughter was entwined with the crackling of the line. 'Sounds like you miss me as much as I miss you.'

'Yes, yes, yes. Oh Ben, I'm lonely without you, I'm so lonely. When will you come?'

His hesitation was loaded; the line's amplified crackling irritating her ear.

'Where are you? The line is so bad.'

There was more hesitation, before he finally replied, 'Italy.'

'What are you doing in Italy? Miss Ruthie would give her right arm to go to Italy to visit the Pope. Are you alone?' she asked.

More hesitation. 'No... can't talk much now, I'll call you later.'

'Who are you with in Italy?' A trace of anger entered her voice.

His hesitation was maddening.

'Claire.'

'And the children?'

'No. Just Claire.'

She hung up, a sob blocking her throat and disappointment fuelling her anger. She knew the cost of this relationship. It shouldn't be a surprise that he had chosen to be in Italy with his wife on some romantic interlude, instead of Jamaica with her. She knew the score, knew he was married. There had been enough time to get out of the situation but she had chosen to stay and now he was in Italy with her, his wife. It really shouldn't matter, it shouldn't be surprising and it shouldn't hurt, but dear God it did. It did.

Kat arrived home alone ahead of the rain that Sunday. Columbus had taken Shadrach to see the town's weekly football match. He was determined that the baby would appreciate the art of football, much to her amusement. Old Man had somehow managed to coax Miss Ruthie to dine with him after Sunday service and they had headed off into town, a smile the size of a Cheshire cat sitting on Jaguar's lips despite the fact that a truck could comfortably pass between them as they strolled.

Kat sat in her chair on the veranda, legs stretched out and crossed at the ankle. Samson, the Labrador watched her thoughtfully with his head resting on his crossed paws. She laughed at such a human trait and it seemed to signal a welcome to him because the next second he was up the steps and settling by her feet. She reached for her pad and pencil on the table beside her but could not add a stroke to the sketch of the ackee tree she was working on. It had been a week since the Blessing, a whole week since she last spoke to Ben. She had no doubt he would have been phoning her but she'd switched off the phone that evening, on learning he was in romantic Italy with his wife. She vowed not to contact him again. It was all still very raw, the pain. The realisation of what she had got herself into without the notion of how she was going to escape.

'Yo, girl!' Kat was jerked out of her thoughts by Rosie, who was dressed in her Sunday Best standing at the gate, under the almond tree. 'You know how long I been standing here watching you? What you considering?' Rosie walked in with her two youngest in tow. The children ran behind Samson who was now heading for the back of the house.

Rosie yelled behind them, 'Watch out for Miss Rootie's vegetable garden round there—she'll kick you to hell and back if you as much as breathe on her carrot or calalloo.' She pulled up the stool to face Kat.

'I bring you some curry chicken.' She held out the plastic container. 'And here's some water from the spring.'

'Thanks.' Kat placed the items on the table.

'Where's Shaddy? Sleeping?'

'No, he's at the ball game with Col.'

'Ball game! A four months' baby? That Englishman is a mad man.'

'He's French, Rosie, don't let him hear you call him English.'

'Foreigners all look the same, can't tell one different from the next. Same white skin that turn red in the sun.'

She looked at Kat's sombre face, no shadow of the contentment that usually occupied it and no smile that would tug her lips apart to reveal the small gap between her teeth.

'What bothering you, Kat? Since the Blessing you been so sad. Tell me.'

Tears bubbled in Kat's eyes and she gulped back the lump travelling the length of her throat. At that moment the skies gave way to the rain and the children came running around the front and underneath the house with Samson scampering behind them to shelter.

'I think maybe I hang my basket higher than I can reach. I thought I was in control, but Miss Ruthie's right, only God have control.'

'We talking parables today?'

Kat looked at Rosie's face, engraved with experience and untold stories and wondered how she bounced back after every love that let her down. Did she have a dream? Had it ever come true and turned out to be something different? How did she let go of the men she desired, wanted, needed, loved? How did she get over pain that dug deep into her heart causing it to bleed utter despair? How did she just carry on running her shop and looking after her kids like nothing had happened? How did she keep on smiling? This was uncharted ground for Kat.

'I think you're incredible, Rosie. So incredible. How do you survive love gone wrong?'

Rosie giggled like an intoxicated school girl. 'You and that posh school your mother sent you to. It teach you to talk like the queen of England or one of them poets.'

Kat's face held no humour. 'How did you get through when it was all over? How did you do it? How long did it take?'

Rosie grew serious. 'I don't live with regrets. When I love, I love and I give it everything and take everything.

And when it goes, I deal with the heartache.' Rosie shrugged her shoulders. 'What bothering you, Kat?'

'I feel empty, Rosie. I thought all I ever needed was my own baby and that love didn't matter. But now I have all I ever thought I wanted, and I want more. I want Ben. I've been trying not to love him too much, I've been fighting it, but I love him and it's all wrong, all wrong. What do I do?'

The rain had simmered to a drizzle and the children and Samson were running around chasing the flapping chickens.

'Stop that!' Rosie bellowed. 'You want Miss Rootie come see you chasing her fowl? She'll boil you alive!' She turned back to Kat. 'You ever tell Ben how you feel?'

Kat shook her head. 'I don't want to pressure him with my demands... but I want him with me and Shaddy and it scares me. I didn't know I was so selfish. Am I cold?'

Initially it had been a great relief as well as disappointment that Ben did not visit during Easter but his promise to be in Jamaica for summer had made up for it. This delay would give her the time to finally break the news to him about his son. He had been so apologetic about his cancelled visit; she could hear the agony in his voice and was touched by guilt at the part of her that was relieved. But phoning him to find out that he was in Italy with his wife gave her a dose of bitter reality which had slowly been strangling her heart.

'No, you're not cold. Just call him and talk,' Rosie advised. 'I can't understand why you say it all wrong, loving the father of your child can't be all wrong, unless him beat you. Him beat you?' Rosie asked, her face filling with concern.

'No,' Kat shook her head vigorously. 'Nothing like that.'

'Why is it all wrong?' Rosie pushed.

Kat felt too ashamed and too hurt. The father of her child was a married man with two children. It had been all so easy in the beginning when all she was anticipating was Mother Cynthy's prediction. Love hadn't been emphasised in the prediction. And now love had proven to be as unpredictable as each day, as passionate as a toddler with his favourite toy and as wild and uncontrollable as a seasonal hurricane.

'How could it have happened without me knowing until it was on top of me?' she turned to ask Rosie. 'It crept up on me and now it's all over me.'

'That's how love is. It only know about satisfying itself, fuck the consequences. The heart wants what the heart wants.'

Kat stared at her friend in amazement. Rosie could sometime make no sense at all, but other times she could be called the mother of all senses.

Kat had known. She could not lie. She knew about his wife and children and how important they were in his life. She could get over the children, but his other love, the love he loved when Kat was not around drove splinters into her. Yet she had brushed away the consequences.

The engine of Columbus' old jeep could be heard some distance away before it reached the front gate. Columbus approached with a proud smile on his face, carrying Shadrach in the baby car seat.

'Hello, Rosie,' he beamed, and turning to Kat, said, 'He enjoyed himself, gurgled and kicked his little legs every time a goal was scored—*un petit footballer ce bébé*... a little footballer this baby.'

It brought a smile to Kat's lips as she reached to take her baby out of the chair. He smiled at his mother in recognition, his arms and legs jerking with excitement and anticipation at being picked up.

'He knows you for sure,' Columbus told her. 'I'll be back in a while, I promised the coach I'd help clear the grounds. Leave some of that curry for me!' he demanded, pointing to the container Rosie had brought. 'And for goodness' sake, turn on your phone so I can get through when I call. Bye.'

'He favours his daddy more and more,' Rosie pointed out, 'them eyes, mouth, but him favour you when he smiles.'

'You remember his daddy's eyes? You only saw him twice.'

'True,' she agreed, 'but who can forget them candy eyes! I don't know what really going on with you but if you love the man just go and be with him. Leave the Meadows.'

After Rosie had left and Shadrach put down for his afternoon nap, Kat finally turned on her mobile phone and immediately it bleeped. Seventy-four missed calls showed. She pressed the return button and phoned Ben.

Twenty-eight

Ben

London

Ben had hurt Kat. He feared that he had also lost her. So when his phone rang late that Sunday evening and her number showed, it was a great relief. Claire and the children were at her mother's for dinner and after barring Auntie Joan's soft plodding around, he was alone.

'Hey you... I thought you'd given up on me.'

'Nearly. I did think about it.'

'A whole week of thinking, huh? Next time can you think with the phone on? Remember the first time I met you and you went AWOL? I nearly went out of my mind. Want to share with me the outcome of a week of thinking?'

'Not over the phone. Are you sure you'll be coming in—'

He cut her short. 'In two months, June 18th, nothing can stop me.'

'How long will you stay?' Her voice was calm and measured but he could sense something deeper.

'A week... About my trip to Italy—'

'Do you seriously think you can explain that?'

His silence told her he couldn't.

'And I can't seriously hold it against you. Are the children okay?'

She always asked about the girls, which he found touching. 'Everyone is fine. How's Miss Ruthie? Is that a baby I hear crying? Whose baby?'

'Yes, it's a baby, his name is Shadrach, we call him Shaddy. I better go see to him.'

'You're babysitting? Okay, call you later... Love you.'

She hesitated, 'We'll see.'

He leaned back in the chair and closed his eyes, whispering silently, *God help me.*

A big surprise would be in store for her when he got to Jamaica. The sale of the three-bedroom house was now complete, the deed and all paperwork in her name. This would make her see how serious he was about their relationship and future together. After she had hung up the phone on him and kept it off for the week, he had felt panicked. It brought it home to him that perhaps what he was offering was not enough. His situation was closing in on him. He felt he was in a tunnel with fast flowing water seeping in and nowhere in sight was there a ledge, a branch of reprieve for him to grasp. Common sense told him it couldn't go on like this forever, but then the heart had never grasped the meaning of common sense.

The A406 at seven in the evening still had its pockets of traffic, brake lights flashing, bumpers kissing, frustration present in the loud honks of horns as people seeking quick ways out switched lanes, yet no-one was getting anywhere too fast. As he drove towards Bubs' flat, he was acutely aware that he didn't want to be alone with his conflicting thoughts hammering for prominence. In truth he had enjoyed Italy, but it didn't stop him thinking how he could have two worlds.

'You know about phoning before turning up on people's doorstep?' Bubs' muscular bare-chested frame blockaded his doorway. Ben pushed past him and headed down the narrow passage that led to the small living room.

'Come in, why don't you.' Bubs used his feet to close the door and followed his friend.

The centre piece of his flat was a large wooden desk that held his computer and hoards of papers and books on landscape gardening. On the magnolia walls hung pictures of a variety of women in different cultural attires.

'You alone?' Ben's head jutted towards the bedroom.

'A little late to be asking that. No, I'm not, Anna's asleep in there.'

'Anna? When did you two get back together?'

'Any time we need to. Wanna drink? Help yourself.'

Bubs flopped down on the brown leather sofa, reaching for the remote control and flicking on the television.

'What's your problem?' Bubs' tone carried irritation.

Ben sat beside him on the sofa, hands clasped. 'I need to get out to Jamaica, Bubs, I need time with Kat. I have to sort something out, you were right, I didn't think far ahead enough.'

'Can't help you there, son, it's your choices and your consequences to face, and you did tell me to mind my own business.'

'Help a brother out.' He lowered his voice, 'I'm

drowning.'

'You ready to end your marriage?'

'I love my wife.'

'Then what's the problem? You have your answer.'

Ben wished it was as simple as that. If life was that straightforward he would not be in this position, where his night and day were near to collision. He felt selfish but lacked the stimulus to correct the situation, hoping, just hoping that things would somehow work themselves out because he didn't have it in him to abandon either of his loves. The thought drove him near to physical pain.

'I'm so far from answers, it's unbelievable. I just need some time alone with Kat so I can work out what's what. I'm going to Jamaica in June because if I don't, my brain will explode.'

'Going to Jamaica is dumb, bro. You're sinking deeper. In a triangle there are no winners, Ben. All players end up hurt, I know you fucking know that much.'

'It doesn't have to be that way. I'm going to do good by both of them. Whatever happens, I'll make sure Claire and the girls don't suffer and Kat won't either. I've got plans in place, Bubs. I've actually bought Kat a house in Meadow View.'

Bubs shook his head despairingly, both hands rising to cup his jaws in dismay.

'It's the right thing to do, Bubs. I feel it. I have to face my responsibilities. I'll find a way to divide my time between here and Jamaica.'

Bubs silence stretched, filling the room to a deafening level while incredulity trickled into his eyes.

'I know I sound like an idiot. I feel like one but I can't reject one and abandon the other. Say something,

Bubs and stop gawping at me like I'm an alien.'

Bubs inhaled deeply, as if preparing for a marathon run. 'Fuck! I mean, what should I say? I ain't never felt that strong about any two women to be that stupid. I thought this Kat thing would eventually pass; you've been carrying her in you for over a year now. I don't know what the fuck to tell you, man. But one thing for sure: you'll eventually have to give her up, you have no responsibility for her.'

Ben looked horrified. 'I can't reject her like that, I–I can't do that to her.'

'So, Claire?'

'I won't abandon my wife and my kids, Bubs.'

Bubs cleared his throat. He slapped Ben firmly on his shoulder. 'Not encouraging you to drink and drive, bro, but have a drink, have fucking two. Because you are one confused motherfucker, if I say so myself.'

Twenty-nine

Kat

Jamaica

Hurricane Jenny was forecast for the month of May, five days after Columbus left for his annual stay in Paris. It was left to Old Man to prepare for the coming storm. He boarded up their house and windows with plywood, secured the roof with straps and clips to the frame structure, trimmed the trees and shrubs around the house and locked up the chickens and Samson in the cage at the back of the house. Miss Ruthie and Kat filled as many bottles and buckets of water as they could and stacked them in crates in the kitchen, and tins of sardines, mackerel, corn beef and packs of rice lined the cupboard shelves. They then settled themselves in the small hallway on mattresses, listening to the radio for updates on the threatening Hurricane Jenny.

By midday the winds were howling, sweeping and whipping everything in its path, hurling the army of dark puffed-up clouds across the sky. The streets were empty of life as the rain began to furiously lash against the shutters. There were times when the house shook, the crack of lightening lit the darkened house and the growling thunder echoed like an angry god. Kat cradled Shadrach in her arms, who was showing signs of frustration at being restricted to such a small space. The turbulence lasted through the night and by dawn the only sign left of Jenny were the fallen trees, turned-over carts and more dangerously, the electrical pylons left lopsided like drunken old men. It took another week before the rain stopped and the sun showed its brilliance once more. Folks in the Meadows always spoke of hurricanes like personal friends and Old Man was no different. 'That Jenny wasn't such a bad girl, she bless us because her eye pass a hundred miles away, saving the town from certain catastrophe.'

As construction began returning the town to normality, Meadow View, up in the suburban hills was the first to have their electricity restored. It took a week longer for the Meadows to be given the same attention and Old Man claimed he knew the reason for this.

'If we had one politician living in our area, we would get electric long time ago!'

Miss Ruthie agreed, 'If we lived in one of them big house up Meadow View, we'd get better treatment. Look how quick their electric come back.'

'They have generators.' Kat's tone was soft and preoccupied. 'Shaddy's father once told me he would buy me a house up there.'

Miss Ruthie looked at Old Man in astonishment. 'You hear her? She say she would leave this house that her daddy worked so hard to build for her.'

Kat laughed, Old Man tried not to, knowing how serious Miss Ruthie was.

'Miss Ruthie, you're so melodramatic. I never said I

would leave this house, I just shared an offer I was made with you. I thought it would make you laugh.'

Miss Ruthie huffed. 'Many a thing said in jest...' she ended knowingly, then whispered to Old Man, 'That foreigner has been sowing ideas in her head.'

*

Her sickle crisis came on suddenly that Wednesday morning. Miss Ruthie always associated a crisis with events happening in Kat's life. Kat knew it was more likely the result of the thought of Ben arriving in less than four weeks. Whatever it was, it brought on a crisis, the first in two years. She was rushed to hospital and given a blood transfusion. As she lay on the hospital bed with her eyes closed and feeling strength returning to her body, she became aware of her mother's presence.

'Where's Shaddy?' she asked.

Miss Ruthie, who had not left her bedside in the four days she was kept in hospital reached out and touched her forehead. 'He with Old Man at the house. I been so worried for you.' A tear rolled down her cheek. 'I been sitting here praying for you. Mother Cynthy say you will be alright. How you feeling, child?'

'Like someone's taken a bat to every part of me.' Her smile was weak.

'Your ears so hard, Kat. If only you—'

'Don't start, Miss Ruthie,' Kat's voice gathered strength.

'I must speak my mind! The truth is by having Shaddy you weaken your body even more. You just couldn't see pass what you want.'

Kat looked at her mother and knew that despite the

love she had for her grandson, she still hadn't forgiven her for having him.

'I don't regret anything, Miss Ruthie.' Her tone was flat, devoid of fight. 'And my body hasn't been weakened by having a baby, that's old wives nonsense.'

'And what about Shaddy's father? He's still in the dark about his child. You don't think he have a right to know he have a five-month-old son? Or is that old wives nonsense? Too many selfish acts, Kat, too many.'

Kat never denied the truth when it confronted her and she could see it. 'You're right about Ben. He should be told about his son and I will tell him.'

'Good. Cause if you don't, the next time he phone you I telling him me-self! That phone of yours been ringing till it nearly mad me, so I answer it and it was him.'

Kat's eyes widened.

'Don't fret, I never tell him nutting about Shaddy. I just say you in the hospital and he start asking as much questions as Nellie Potato. I tell him you sick, but not serious. Columbus call too and I tell him. He send some money through Western Union and I pick it up, God bless Columbus.'

'What did Ben say?' The crisis had arrived so suddenly that she had no time to turn off her phone.

'He just ask what wrong with you.'

'And you told him?'

'Yes. I don't know why you didn't tell him before.'

'What did he say?'

'Nutting. Just want to know if you alright and when you coming home.'

Kat sighed. She could not keep the charade up any longer. It was time for Ben to know the truth about everything. It was long overdue.

Rosie arrived later the following day to find Kat sitting on the veranda with her sketch pad blank. There was no sun or breeze and the air felt close and stuffy.

'You survive Jenny, eh!' Rosie beamed.

'Did you suffer any damage? Old man says we were lucky because the eye passed us,' Kat responded.

'God was with me, my little house never lose as much as a board and Nellie Potato's big fancy concrete house lose the roof. There's a God! I know Miss Rootie not in or you would still be in bed like sickness itself.' She laughed as she climbed the steps to seat herself.

'She's taken Shaddy to visit the Pastor, Old Man came to collect her.'

'They growing strong, eh! Rumour have it them courting. I went in the post office yesterday and Nellie Potato asking me nuff questions about Miss Rootie's bizness. I keep my mouth shut and run out a that shop so quick 'cause I fear Miss Rootie cuss me to hell and back.'

Kat laughed. 'You know she would.'

'You heard from Candy Eyes?'

'He's coming next month.' She sighed, 'When we were teenagers I could only dream about having a baby. I never thought I would, not with Miss Ruthie always reminding me about how it would kill me and me half-believing her. When you kept having babies year after year, I thought you were the luckiest girl alive. You and I have always been able to talk to each other, and most of the time I've felt safe telling you things.'

Rosie was her friend and she loved her dearly but Kat

had not told her the truth about Ben. Her shop on the beach was a hangout for locals from the Meadows and a beehive for gossip, second only to Nellie Potato in the post office. Kat knew Rosie would not intentionally let it slip, but by her own admission she was not good at holding secrets.

'What is it?' Rosie asked.

Kat fidgeted with her fingers, bit her bottom lip and sighed again.

Rosie peered at her, puzzled. 'You want to talk about it?'

Kat sighed once more. 'Your mouth is not your own, Rose-Lilly Thompson.'

Rosie laughed, opening her arms up to the sky. 'So, you want to tell me something that can't go no further?' She clapped her hands, then rubbed them together with glee. Kat looked at her with severe displeasure.

'You always take serious things for a joke, Rosie, forget I even said anything.'

Rosie giggled, covering her mouth as Kat's disapproving glare held on. 'Okay,' she said, trying to stifle the laughter. 'It's just sometimes you can sound so much like Miss Rootie. Lighten up, nuh! I swear, I give you my word that what you tell me will go no further.'

Kat's dubious look kept Rosie's mouth promising. Rosie put a hand to her heart. 'God believe me, if I say anything, may he strike me down dead.' Then stilling the laughter completely she took Kat's hand. 'I know I love gossiping, and I can only keep a secret for two days max, but if you really need me to stay dumb about this, you have my word, on my life!'

'Good, because if this goes beyond you and me, our

friendship done! I would never speak to you again, ever,' Kat warned and Rosie nodded in excited agreement.

'Ben, he's... he's married. And he has two daughters.' Kat squirmed, watching closely for Rosie's disappointment. She knew Rosie held her in high regard and was impressed by her schooling and education. This high expectation held by folks in the Meadows of educated children was unrealistic and pressurising, as far as Kat was concerned. Yet examining her own feelings about Ben, about loving a married man, she felt she had let a lot of people down, including herself, but still held firm to the belief that fate was the master.

A frown appeared across Rosie's brow. 'How long you know this?' she asked, her voice giving nothing away.

'Not at the beginning, but before he went back home.'

'No wonder you say it wrong to love your baby daddy, you knew he was married,' Rosie spoke slowly, her eyes collecting disapproval as the realisation hit her. 'What you want me to say?'

Kat felt the threat of tears. Rosie was angry with her. 'You think I did wrong?'

Rosie sucked on her teeth. 'You asking me these questions now? Why you never ask when you find out?'

'I–I... It was a confusing time for me, Rosie. I'm even more confused now.'

Rosie heaved. 'All that education... and for what? You know this can't work, don't? You must know he'll never leave his wife for you? What was going on in your mind?' she barked.

Kat felt under attack. 'Mother Cynthy's prediction. I thought once I had the baby I would feel... well I thought everything would be alright, my life would be complete.'

Rosie shook her head gravely. 'You live too much in your own universe.'

Kat stared ahead miserably.

'What will you do now? He's coming soon... so what? You going to ask him to leave his wife and pickney? How you have so much education and you don't know married men don't leave their wives for mistresses.'

'I'm not his mistress, don't say that.'

'Then what are you? You slept with a married man, you have him pickney, you're not his wife, you're his mistress, his mistress. Don't fool yourself. What are you hoping for?'

With a violent shake of her head, Kat stood up, fighting to control the urge to burst into tears. She wasn't sure of anything anymore. The only thing she knew for certain was she wanted Ben and she knew that wasn't fair to him.

Thirty

Ben

London

Ben was worried. He didn't understand why Kat would keep her illness a secret. Especially an illness that hospitalised her. He didn't know much about sickle cell, until he Googled the information. All he knew about the illness before was that Bubs had a daughter who carried the sickle cell trait, which caused her little to no problem, except sometimes in the winter Bubs would mention she was off school with joint pains.

He walked into the bedroom and stood by the door, watching Claire discretely as she slipped into her matching lilac underwear, freshly showered and moisturised from head to toe. Her long hair fell in ringlets and she leaned forward to look in the mirror, adding blueberry lipstick to her pouting lips.

'You really are beautiful.' Ben suddenly felt tearful.

Claire turned around and smiled temptingly. 'You think?' She placed both hands on her hip and gave a little wiggle. 'You really think I'm still beautiful?' She walked into his arms and he drew her in, holding her tight.

'Yes,' he replied with a husky voice.

'I think I'm spectacular too, only I hate the scar left after the ectopic.'

'It hardly shows, Claire. There's not one part of your body that satisfies you... why?'

'That's how us girls are.'

'All of you?'

'Well, name one woman who's satisfied with all she has... you can't because she doesn't exist.' She stepped out of his arms and reached for her dress, turning her back to slip into it. 'Zip me up; we're going to be late.'

He was taking her to their favourite tapas restaurant in the heart of Soho.

He inhaled her as he zipped her dress. 'You smell divine.'

She smiled, turning around to snuggle in his arms. They kissed, softly at first, picking up passion. He loved her. He loved his wife. God, this was complicated.

'You sure you want this Spanish food?' He was kissing her neck, travelling towards her breast.

'Are we going to be able to go someplace before you go off to Jamaica? Maybe a weekend in Paris? I think we should have more "us" time,' she giggled.

He loved when she laughed.

'We only just came back from Italy a few months ago,' he pointed out.

'That's my point. Between you, me and these walls, Taylor confided in me that she and Leon might not make it. She says he's been having an affair. It's so sad, Benny, they've been together since school. They did marry young but so did we. They have three kids, we have two. I want us to keep our marriage fresh; you know, go off sometimes and just be Ben and Claire, nobody's parents.'

'Whatever you want, but let's not talk about your friends or compare them to us. Please.' His heart was beating uncomfortably fast. He released her and she kept talking, 'Mummy and Helen said the same. Helen's been coaching Taylor, told her to pack Leon's things in black bin bags and leave them on the doorstep with a note and—'

Ben stopped her chatter with his finger to her lips. 'Promise me that you'll never take advice from your mother or Helen... they've both got issues. Now strip—'

'No way, I'm starving, let's go,' she was laughing.

'Are you choosing tapas over me?' He pulled her close from behind, then started to unzip her dress.

She did a full turn out of his arms, laughing. 'I'm looking forward to a prawn and piquillo tortilla, I'm going to stuff my face... then I'll have you for dessert. How do I look?' She twirled.

His mobile rang. He took it out of his pocket and glanced at the screen. It was Kat. He placed it back into his pocket. His heart rocked.

'Beautiful, Claire. You're beautiful.'

As they drove out of the driveway, one of Professor Faintheart's favourite Shakespearean sayings from Ben's childhood bounced around in his head. "Oh what a tangled web we weave, when first we practice to deceive."

Thirty-One
Miss Ruthie
Jamaica

Miss Ruthie sighed heavily with every few steps she took as she showered corn to the pecking chickens. She called out to Kat to make haste to help. She knew the morning ahead would be glorious but that by afternoon the clouds would swell and sprinkle its contents on the dry baked earth. That was the month of June in the Meadows. It involved hot mornings, wet afternoons and cool nights.

Kat came out of the house looking tired, still in her dressing gown and slippers, her hair covered under a colourful scarf. The newest feature to their yard was tied to the front gate, under the almond tree; Charmaine the brown and white heifer, a gift from Old Man. Charmaine provided the milk for many of the folks in the Meadows and their front yard was now busier than usual in the mornings. Old Man came early to milk her and placed the bucket on ice blocks until it was all sold, which was often before the sun split the sky. Rumours circled though, spread like butter on hot bread by Nellie Potato that something untoward was going on between Ruthie and Old Man. It was upsetting for Miss Ruthie and it took all her self-control not to give Nellie Potato a mouthful of words that would hurt her dead mama six feet under. Ruthie had gained strength from Old Man over the months and their friendship had warmed and given her peace that served as an armour against gossip.

'I taking Charmaine up on the green now,' Old Man told Miss Ruthie after packing ice around the bucket of milk.

'Make sure you don't let her graze on Farmer Tom's grass, I don't want him or Nellie Potato making no claim on my dumb animal!'

He chuckled as he untied the cow and led her away, passing Nellie Potato at the gate.

The tight-face Nellie nodded, a smirk easily sliding across her lips.

'Morning, Jaguar.'

Old Man returned the salutation without a smile and strolled leisurely along, Charmaine in tow.

'Morning, Kat, how is the baby?' asked Nellie, walking through the opened gate and into the yard.

'He's fine, still sleeping.' Kat's tone was flippant.

'I'll take half dozen tomato, onions and two avocados... oh, and if you can fill this bottle with milk... Morning, Miss Rootie, everything fine with you?' Her comment as usual was laced with an underlying tease served with sarcasm to maximise effect.

Ruthie responded, 'Everything is good—praise Sweet Jesus for he is merciful.' She continued feeding the chickens, her lips set in a grim line. She thought Nellie Potato would leave swiftly owing to her obvious mood, but she hung around like a hungry dog in anticipation of food, despite her milk and provisions firmly tucked under her arms.

'Was there something else, Miss Nellie?' Kat enquired.

Nellie Potato looked at her with a know-it-all expression. 'I believe I have everything I need. See you in church Sunday, Miss Rootie. Maybe you can get the heathen Old Man to come and give thanks to his Creator. How is the father of your son doing, Kat? He been to see his child yet? It really look bad for you... being left unmarried with a child to raise on your own, very sinful.'

Miss Ruthie's head jerked up, and she immediately saw the storm coming. The thunder that darkened her daughter's face, the lightening that flashed in her eyes and finally the unleashing of the flood of words that gushed like a broken dam from her mouth.

'Who is more heathen than you?' Kat spewed, taking a threatening step to face Nellie Potato. 'You're the one who needs saving. You're the most malicious, nosey, back-biting sinner to ever walk on God's earth! You need to go mind your own business and keep an eye on your woman-chasing-husband and don't come sniffing round here in the hope of finding gossip to spread!'

Nellie's jaws opened and closed like a fish out of water. It was a first, no sound emitting from a mouth so used to words. She stood rooted in astonishment and clothed in mounting anger. Only it couldn't match the anger that confronted her in Kat's frosted eyes. Miss Ruthie had stopped her busying and now stood in silence, her head bouncing from her daughter to Nellie Potato.

'I–I–I never been so insulted in my entire life! I know you from the womb of your mother—I knew your father more than you ever will! I am a Christian—a true

248

follower of Lord Jesus! How dare you talk to me like that!' Her voice quivered.

Kat was not to be perturbed. 'True Christians don't take part in malicious gossip. They don't condemn people for being happy, for loving another human outside of being married.'

'The sanctity of marriage is right in the sight of our Lord! I will never go against it and all who do are sinners who will burn in hell!'

'And what about old married men seducing young girls, spending their wives' money on them... like your husband does with your hard-earned money. Will he burn in hell too? And what about you who turn a blind eye to all his sins, doesn't that put you in hell also?'

Nellie Potato clutched a handful of her blouse, almost choking herself as she looked at the silent Miss Ruthie for some form of support.

'Tell me you didn't know! Go on, lie and tell me you didn't know your husband seduced Ma Gem's simple daughter, made her all sorts of promises and left her pregnant. Tell me young Tin-Tin doesn't look the image of Farmer Tom and a handful of your children! Tell me so that I can condemn your lying soul to hell! And maybe if you wasn't so wicked, God wouldn't have let Jenny take off your roof.'

'Blasphemy!' Nellie Potato squealed. 'Blasphemy!'

'The truth is an offence, it is not a sin!' Kat screamed back.

'I'm only trying to do my Christian duty and prevent your soul from going to hell. You prefer, heaven or hell?'

'I have friends in both those places, so worry more about your soul, and if you need an extra soul to fret about, then your husband's is a good place to start.'

By now a small crowd had been attracted by the raised voices and stood with blatant curiosity outside the gate. Nellie Potato turned on her heels, forgetting the arthritic hips and knees she often complained about and pushed her way through the group.

Finally Kat dared to turn and look at her mother expecting to see recrimination and condemnation.

'You should really respect your elders, Kat,' Miss Ruthie's mouth said, but from her eyes shone admiration. For the first time in years, since Kat graduated from university, Ruthie felt that familiar feeling of a mother's pride.

After church that Sunday morning, Miss Ruthie didn't change out of her white cotton lace dress, crisp white hat with the pink ribbon and Italian pink scarf that draped her shoulders—the one Old Man Jaguar had given her. She sat on the veranda, with her customary brown paper bag filled with rice grains, humming. There was no sun but it was humid and sticky and she fanned herself with a folded old newspaper.

'You want a drink, Miss Ruthie?' Kat opened the door holding out a glass packed with ice and homemade lemonade. Miss Ruthie smiled and took the glass thankfully.

'Just what I need.' She gulped down the cold liquid and handed the empty glass back to Kat. 'More would be good,' she said.

'Are you not getting undressed out of your church clothes?' Kat asked.

'No, Old Man say he taking me to see that Father Marshall from America—he's a wise man of God and giving a sermon.'

Kat's eyes opened in surprise. 'Old Man getting religious on you?'

Ruthie laughed. 'I tell him Nellie Potato call him a heathen and that make him so mad. I tell him how you cuss her out, how she run from the house like Lucifer out of heaven.'

Miss Ruthie's laughter rang out as Kat disappeared into the house with the glass, talking at the top of her voice, 'I don't regret my words to nosey Nellie Potato.'

'She hasn't step foot back since, although she sent her granddaughter, Su-Anne to purchase her provisions, with her flat face, like when cow shit pon broad stone.' Miss Ruthie quickly made the sign of the cross for her sinful words.

It took a while for Miss Ruthie to register Mother Cynthy standing at the gate, worry occupying her face. Mother Cynthy stood perfectly still for a moment, even after Ruthie had beckoned to her. She balanced the basket on her head before opening the gate and stepping in.

'Morning, Mother Cynthy,' Ruthie beamed.

The old woman walked slowly up the steps, removing the basket and placing it by her feet.

'Morning, Miss Rootie, you going somewhere?'

Ruthie nodded. 'Old Man taking me to see an American priest, him giving a sermon. You want to come with us?'

Mother Cynthy's expression mocked horror. 'No, no, no, the Old Man wouldn't want that! You go enjoy yourself—you deserve it.'

Kat emerged with the filled glass which she handed

to her mother.

'Hi, Mother Cynthy, would you like a drink?'

'Yes, some water full of ice will do.'

Kat disappeared back inside the house, humming to herself.

'Everything alright, Mother Cynthy? You look like you get premonition. Is Kat alright?' asked Ruthie, frowning.

'Yes, Yes. You worry too much. Just enjoy yourself with the Old Man and stop fussing.'

'You sure? Only you have that look... the one that say you know more than you revealing.'

Kat's presence interrupted them. 'Here's your water,' she said, handing the glass to Mother Cynthy.

'Thank you. How's master Shaddy?' Mother Cynthy asked between sips.

'Sleeping. He always comes back sleeping after Miss Ruthie takes him to church.'

They were deep in conversation when Old Man arrived dressed in the light blue safari suit and yellow shirt he had worn to church earlier. His polished brown shoes and brown feathered hat made him seem more dressed for a party.

He tipped his hat. 'Wishing you a good day, Mother Cynthy, Miss Kat.'

Mother Cynthy smiled warmly, as though she was greeting a good friend.

'You looking mighty dapper, Old Man. Jus' make sure Miss Rootie enjoy herself... and you too, make sure you have the time of your life.'

Old Man laughed. 'Is the first time in my life that you say a decent word to me, write it down, Miss Rootie, write down this day.'

Miss Ruthie looked dubiously at Mother Cynthy, her brows knitting together in confusion but she stayed silent.

'Enjoy your day and don't keep my mother out too late, Old Man,' Kat teased. She kissed them both, touched to see them looking so happy and at ease with each other.

Miss Ruthie looked at Old Man's profile as they strolled along. He had taken her hand and linked through his arms and she had allowed it with no protest. She could see how proud and happy he looked and for the first time she was not concerned with what Nellie Potato or the other town folks would think. Kat's confrontation with Nellie had saturated the whole Meadows and many more people were pleased about it than displeased. It was the topic of the moment, in bars, on street corners, in the barber shop and hairdressing salons. They even congratulated Miss Ruthie, as if it was actually her that had finally told the nosey post mistress about herself.

They walked to the end of the lane where they took a taxi into the town centre to Hotel Panama where Father Marshall, the Roman Catholic priest from America would deliver his sermon.

Waiting for the homily to begin, Miss Ruthie felt very important. She was seated among the wealthy of the Meadows, some of them white people. Oh how she wished Nellie Potato could see her now.

After the four-hour sermon, the hotel provided drinks in tall elegant glasses and bite-size food on dainty flower-patterned plates—food so small you could stuff at least ten of the little pastries into your mouth at the same time and still have space for more. This would not fill her stomach, but she was looking forward to letting Nellie Potato know. It surprised her how well Old Man spoke with the white folks, how they all seemed to know and like him. The feeling that grew within her as she watched him talking and laughing with them made tears come to her eyes. She had always seen Old Man as a rum drinker not to be taken serious. Why, he seemed only to enjoy rum and preferred it to coming to Sunday worship and didn't seem as though he had a religious bone in his body. Yet here he was talking with these posh white folks and the rich black folks about the Bible and what a good sermon Father Marshall had delivered. Her heart expanded with so much pride she thought she would burst. Where was Nellie Potato to see this?

'You alright, Miss Rootie?' Old Man asked after returning to her side.

She smiled. 'Yes. The sermon was one of the best I ever hear... thank you for bringing me, Old Man.'

The smile that spread itself across his face, the twinkle that filled his eyes as he looked at her caused a warmth to engulf her that she had never felt before. She blushed and turned her head away.

'I wouldn't think of bringing anyone but you—you is my world, Miss Rootie and anything I can do to make you happy, make you smile with me, I will do it.'

'It be good if you would put away your rum and answer to the call of Sweet Jesus, Old Man. When the time is right and the Lord come for you, I want you going to heaven,' she told him, her hand reaching out to straighten his bowtie.

'This is as much as you going to get, Miss Rootie. I love the Lord no less than you, but I must show it in my own way. I intend to go to heaven when the time right. Come now, I book a table so we can have dinner.'

'Here?' Miss Ruthie's eyes opened with joy, her mouth dropping in surprise and pleasure.

'Yes. I chose that table in the corner by the door so we can get some of the breeze.'

They were led by a waiter who was dressed all in white, looking so immaculate that Miss Ruthie felt like royalty. He pulled out the chair for her to sit down and she felt she could faint with all the attention. The food, she thought, was not as seasoned as she would have liked, but if this was how the rich ate, then she could do it also.

'You like it?' Old Man asked eagerly.

She nodded. Even if the food tasted bland, she could still say she dined at the posh Panama Hotel where all the rich people go. She could tell them how the waiter had waited on her and pulled out the chair for her to sit on. She would be proud to tell them how Old Man could talk good to white folks who listened to him like he was one of the wise men from the Bible.

'How much this cost? You not breaking your pocket are you?'

'Oh, Miss Rootie, don't concern yourself 'bout my pocket, I just want to know you enjoying it.'

'Maybe,' she smiled.

'In all the years I know you, I never hear you say yes or no.' He laughed, his eyes full of such warmth and love she felt breathless. She wanted to reach across the table and touch the smile on his lips but felt that would be going too far in public.

'I want to be bold enough to ask you a question... but I fear you cuss me.'

Ruthie's soft laughter was filled with invitation.

'Would you consider becoming my wife, Miss Rootie? You would make me the happiest man alive. I know the answer but it won't make me stop asking the question over and over—'

'Maybe, Old Man.' Her response stopped him in mid-sentence.

He looked at her in amazement. 'Maybe as in yes? Or Maybe as in no?'

'Maybe... as in maybe.'

For a long moment he sat staring at her, the smile filling his face, his eyes bright with the gathering water. He reached for her hands and kissed them. He stood up.

'Dance with me, Miss Rootie... come, let me dance you.'

'But there's no music, Old Man... you losing your senses or what!'

'I'll hum and we dance.' He waved her objections to one side and took her in his arms, slowly waltzing her as she blushed at the smiles they were receiving from the other guests. He was humming that song, *When a Man Loves a Woman*, and it wasn't sounding too bad, she admitted inside.

'She's going to be my bride,' he shouted, much to Miss Ruthie's embarrassment.

The whole restaurant cheered, their noise becoming the music Old Man waltzed her, spinning her around until she was dizzy with laughter and the closeness of him.

'I love you, Miss Rootie, I always have,' he whispered in her ear. 'I have some money save, I want to take you to Italy, so you can see the Pope in Vatican City with you own eyes.'

Miss Ruthie's head rested on Old Man's shoulders. He smelled of baby lotion and lavender, with no scent of the faint waft of rum that usually followed him.

She was going to marry Old Man and go Italy to see the Pope. It had been many decades since she had felt this happy and couldn't wait to share the news with the whole Meadows.

Thirty-two

Miss Ruthie

Miss Ruthie was predictable. Her mornings, afternoons, evenings and her Sundays through to Saturdays consisted pretty much of the same routine. She ate at the same times each day, she worked the same set hours daily, went to bed at the same time and got up at the same time. If there was ever a creature of habit competition, Miss Ruthie would take first prize. However, that Monday morning when Kat got up at the usual 5am to assist with the setting up of the shop for the day's sale, Miss Ruthie remained in bed. Concerned, Kat walked along the small hallway, still cloaked in darkness, which led to Miss Ruthie's room. She swept the curtain that acted as a door to one side and gently called her mother.

'I'm right here,' Miss Ruthie replied, a smile softening her face in the dim light of daybreak. She was sat up in bed, propped up by two large pillows behind her back, the Bible on her lap. Daybreak was trying to make an impression on the still dark skies, and the noise of the morning, the cock crowing, cut through the tranquil air. Kat moved to sit on her mother's bed and felt compelled to get under the thin sheet where she could sit closer.

It had been a long time since she had done this. It used to be a regular thing on Saturday and Sunday evenings, Kat sitting and snuggling up to her mother and them listening to the World Service together. Miss Ruthie had never liked the idea of a television and as a child if Kat wanted to watch a programme, she would go and sit around Old Man's house and fiddle with the aerial on his television set until some kind of picture showed. She waited until the end of her university years before she bought her own television, which she placed in her room and actually hardly ever switched on because the reception was so bad.

'Is something wrong, Miss Ruthie? Why are you not up getting the provisions ready? Are you feeling ill?' Miss Ruthie felt Kat's hand on her brow.

'I'm not sick at all child, not at all.'

'Then why are you still in bed past 5am?'

Miss Ruthie closed the bible and placed it on the small side table beside her bed. Clasping her hands together, she sighed.

'I'm not working today... not today.'

'Why?'

'I do something and I want you to be happy about it.'

'Are you happy about it?'

'Maybe.'

Kat laughed. 'Then I'm happy. Now tell me, what am I happy about?'

'I tell Old Man I'll marry him.'

Kat could not hide her surprise. It left her speechless and motionless. Miss Ruthie herself could hardly believe what she had agreed to last night. Maybe it was the intoxication of the evening. Seeing Father Marshall, then being introduced to all them rich people, being wined and dined and finally, dancing in front of all those people who clapped and looked so happy for them. Old Man had truly swept her off her feet. And what astonished her more was that she felt no different this morning. She was glad she had accepted his offer of marriage. She was looking forward to being his wife.

'Of course I know he will never change his ways. He will always be Old Man... love to drink his rum and play dominoes. I don't think I can turn him to Sweet Jesus my way, but he love the Lord in him own way. He's a good man... a fine, fine man... and he's been there for so long, always helping me... helping us.'

Miss Ruthie felt her daughter's arm around her. 'This is such good news, Miss Ruthie. I'm happy for you, and Old Man is like a father to me. When will the wedding be? Can I be a bridesmaid?'

Miss Ruthie patted her daughter's hand. 'Soon, then we going to foreign, to Italy to see the Pope and the Vatican. I never even leave Jamaica in my life and I only ever travel to the city once and that's before you born. Now Old Man taking me... I going to fly in a plane and see the clouds.'

By midday Miss Ruthie was checking the time every few minutes. Old Man hadn't come around to milk Charmaine yet and she could only think that he had gone home and drunk too much rum and was now worse for wear. The breakfast she had prepared for him was long cold and she turned customers away because no shop or milk was available that day. Finally she could no longer sit and wait for him. She dressed in her yellow cotton dress, donned her straw hat and wore a shawl over her shoulders, fully aware she looked as though she was going somewhere special. Should she be seen going to Old Man's the rumours it would cause. But for once in her life she did not care. She was soon to be Mrs Ivan Price, wife of Old Man, and she was looking forward to being his, cooking for him and making sure he laid off the rum drinking and came to church at least once a month.

He lived halfway up Meadow Mountains, where the dirt turned red and the air was cool, so cool that the locals thought it cold and wore extra clothing to venture there. Miss Ruthie had not been to Meadow Mountains in many years and it was even more years since she had seen Old Man's house. Her dear departed husband used to go regularly to play dominoes with him and occasionally she went to the mountains with Mother Cynthy to fill her bottles with the spring water that sprouted from the ground like a celebration of nature and which was said to have healing properties.

She chartered a taxi to take her up to the mountains, pleasantly reminding the driver that she wanted to get there in one piece so he should take the winding road and the corners with more consideration. The taxi came to a halt where the red dirt road turned to rocks, stones and pebbles. From there she followed the stony path that would lead her to Old Man's house. She was surprised to see a small group of men and women outside and wondered if their presence was as a result of Old Man spreading the word about the coming wedding. The group turned to watch her and she smiled because she was going to show them that she was proud of her husband-to-be, despite his rum drinking and what they may consider his unholy ways. As she neared them, she became puzzled. They all seemed to be watching her with sympathy, mumbling under their breath words she could not hear. They parted the way, making a path for her to walk up to the house. Nellie Potato had been right, Old Man had built an extension and the veranda showed signs of being newly renovated.

Their mumbling became hushed and they were viewing her with such sadness, such sympathy that she wanted to shout and tell them not to pity her because she was going to marry a good man, a man of the Lord in his own way.

'We should pray,' she heard a woman's voice say.

'He's strong, but no man is this strong.'

A cold, clammy hand gripped her heart and she realised it was pounding heavily. She could make no sense of what they were saying and hurriedly pushed past them up the few steps on to the veranda and through the opened door. She was startled to see Dr Mattie coming out of a room, her face grim.

'Miss Ruthie, come, let's take a seat—'

'Not now, Dr Mattie, I come to see Old Man—'

The doctor grabbed her hand gently. 'Miss Ruthie, I'm sorry to say he's had a stroke. He's unconscious but the ambulance is on its way—'

Ruthie did not hear the end of Dr Mattie's sentence. She hurried into the room and there was Old Man asleep, propped up by pillows. He had on red striped pyjamas and his left leg was slightly bent. The room looked as though it had been recently painted and a picture of a black Christ, his hand folded across his heart hung over the bed. She smiled. He did love the Lord in his own way.

'Old Man,' she whispered, 'Old Man, what you doing laying in bed playing sick? I make breakfast for you and Charmaine need milking.'

He stirred. She moved closer to the bed and touched his feet, they were warm. She gingerly walked around to the side of the bed where his turned head was facing. His eyes were closed and he was smiling. She bent over and touched the smile on his lips, made lop-sided by the stroke. She sat on the bed. Then she laid down beside him, looking at his smiling face. He still smelled like baby lotion and lavender.

'Old Man... Old Man, don't you leave me. No, don't do that. Don't leave me, not now. I want to cook for you, I want to be your wife... don't go. I can't live in a world without you there.' Tears fell down her cheeks.

She was inconsolable as the paramedics came and carried Old Man into the ambulance. Her face had lost its glow, its softness and roundness was now replaced by gauntness and her whole body seemed to have withered and died in minutes. She ached with anxiety and for moments was angry with her Maker. How could he have put her through this again? Did she not deserve to have love, to sleep beside love and have it hold her in its arms? How cruel this was. Was it her punishment for not marrying Old Man sooner? He'd been asking for so many years and had she not cared about what people would say, she would have married him many moons ago. Her dear, dear love. She knew that if Old Man was to die, then she would die too.

Thirty-three
Miss Ruthie

Kat sat on the veranda before her mother, trying to spoon-feed her through tightly pursed lips her favourite cornmeal porridge.

'Miss Ruthie, won't you eat something... please. If you don't start eating you'll die of starvation!'

Tears gathered in Miss Ruthie's eyes until it could no longer contain the pool and they spilled out and rolled down her face.

'Oh Miss Ruthie, what shall I do with you?' Kat placed the bowl of porridge on the table and wiped the tears away with her hands. 'Why won't you eat? Not eating won't make Old Man any better.'

Miss Ruthie remained silent. This silence was her way of punishing herself for wasting all those years she could have been Old Man's wife. She could still feel his arms around her, waltzing with her and humming in her ear, showing her off to all those white and rich folks. See his smiling face, his twinkling eyes that could house so much mischief. If she could only have one more day with him. One more waltz. If only she had accepted his proposal, now it was all too late and too painful. She started sobbing.

'Oh Miss Ruthie,' Kat cried in despair. 'He'll get better, I know he will. Old Man won't leave you.'

Miss Ruthie wished she could believe that but with each day he lay in that coma things were looking worse.

The scurrying of the chicken caused them both to look up as the gate opened and Mother Cynthy walked in. Miss Ruthie suddenly remembered she had seen something in Mother Cynthy's eyes that day Old Man took her to the Sermon.

'Morning, Miss Rootie, still not using your tongue?' Mother Cynthy said. As usual she placed her laden basket by her feet and sat down.

'I'm glad you've come, Mother Cynthy. I have to go feed Shaddy. Will you try and convince my mother to eat before she drops dead? There's her porridge.' Kat pointed to the bowl on the table.

'She'll eat when she good and ready, no-one can't force her,' Mother Cynthy said, looking gently at Miss Ruthie. 'You breaking Old Man's heart, Miss Rootie. He don't want you doing this to yourself.'

Miss Ruthie watched her oldest friend unsmiling and with sparks of accusations emitting from her eyes.

'I know you vex with me... mad like a spitting cobra. You think I know Old Man was going to have the stroke, but I didn't know it was Old Man, I did think it was you.'

Miss Ruthie's brow met in a frown.

'You and I know that sometimes visions don't walk straight. I think it was you and I was nice to Old Man cause I know he would be sad... He's sad to see you like this.'

Suddenly they were distracted by a commotion at the

gate. Mama Gem came chasing Samson with a broom and the dog squeezed himself under the gate to avoid a bashing and ran onto the veranda by Miss Ruthie's side.

'Miss Rootie, I know you still worrying about Old Man, but please keep your animal out of my garden. I spend plenty money on my rosebush and I will mash him head to pieces if him sniff round again. I can't understand why he come just to pull at my roses and run like that, Samson never trouble my garden before but if him do it again... it's war between me and him!'

Miss Ruthie showed no concern. In the past she would be ready for a war of words over any threat made to Samson, but now she was just too tired, too old and broken.

Kat came out with Shadrach in her arms. 'What's that Samson have in his mouth?' she asked, pointing. Reluctantly Miss Ruthie looked down. Her heart stood still. Then she felt a new breath enter her lungs and she started breathing heavily.

'Miss Ruthie, are you alright? What's wrong? Mother Cynthy, do something!' Kat cried.

'She alright,' Mother Cynthy assured. 'She just decide to live again.'

Ruthie's hand went out to remove the item from Samson's mouth. It was one of Old Man's gardening gloves. She smiled through her tears. This was a good omen. Old Man had been looking for that glove for many weeks, refusing to buy a new one because he said it would turn up. And he was right. She somehow knew he would be alright.

Thirty-four

Ben

The warm gust of air was his first welcome back onto Jamaican soil. As he came out of Montego Bay airport he smiled up to the heavens. In a few minutes he would see Kat again, hold her, fall into her eyes and taste her lips. He hastened his steps as he caught sight of her standing to the side of the door by arrivals. Her hair had grown and was free from its usual ponytail, left wild like an unruly child just out of a tantrum—it was becoming. She wore a fitted white dress, his favourite colour on her, with large black buttons down the front. Her eyes held his from a distance and she pulled him in until he stood before her, a carnival of emotions whirling inside.

'Hey, sweet girl.'

'Ben.'

She fell against him and he pulled her close, inhaling her. The urge to kiss was overpowering and he gently pulled her by the hair until her head tilted back. He kissed her, soft small kisses until the urge expanded like bread in water. The airport was a place for greetings and farewells. It certainly wasn't unusual to see emotions on parade and even if it was, he didn't give a damn; she was real and after all these months, finally in his arms.

In the taxi she sunk against him, her silence and the underlying current of her passion hot and pregnant with anticipation. A heavy seductive mist clouded her eyes and parted her lips deliciously causing him to consciously control his breathing and the urge to part her legs and take her there and then in the taxi.

'Oh Ben, I'm so glad you're here. Life is so short.' She buried her face in his neck. 'I don't know what I would do if something were to happen to you.'

'Are you okay?' He became concerned. 'Why say such a thing?'

'Someone very special to me... us, Miss Ruthie and I... he had a stroke. He's on the mend now, but it's been hard.'

'I'm sorry, baby, so sorry.'

'We shouldn't waste time because we won't get it back. Hold me.'

He was given the same room in the guest house in Meadow View, and the first thing Kat did was close the blinds so darkness was complete. The familiarity made it all the more welcoming and they fell into each other's arms, loosening and peeling off clothing until at last their bodies met like magnet to steel. Hours later they fell asleep, bodies and limbs so tangled that had it not been the difference in the shades of their skins, it would have been impossible to see where they each began and ended.

The crashing sea against the cliffs was the background melody of the sounds that drifted through the opened window of their room, rousing Ben out of his passion-filled stupor. Beside him soundly sleeping, was his very own sleeping beauty, the blackness of her hair stark against the whiteness of the cotton pillow. He pulled her close again and began to extract soft moans and movements from her aroused body. He smiled and hoped this moment would last a life time.

They eventually had to get up to eat and attend to nature's call. They took breakfast in bed and fed each other and ate off each other's lips, bodies and hands.

'I've been waiting for this moment for so long, it seems. Have you missed me, girl? You been miserable without me?'

'Yes, you know that. But we've got some talking to do.'

'Yeah, I know—me first. Let's shower and dress, there's something I want to show you.'

'And there's someone I want to introduce to you.'

The taxi was parked at the front of the guest house, under a Blue Mahoe tree, the driver making the most of its shade from the broad leaves. Ben held the door of the car opened as Kat got inside, sliding to the other side to make space for him. It was a short drive from the guest house to Meadow View, an affluent area situated in the hills above the Meadows, and where the majority of houses belonged to foreigners or returnees; people who had made a life abroad in America or Europe and had bought holiday or retirement homes right there. Ben paid the driver and directed the taxi to pull up outside a detached house, as all the houses were and which had two palm trees on either side of the black iron gates. The shutters were green against the cream of the stone-built townhouse and matched the luscious green of the front lawn. There to the right of the lawn was a garden patch with roses and a group of baby's breath surrounding them.

'Who lives here?' she enquired, confused. 'Look, they have baby's breath.'

'Let's look inside.' He took her hand and led her firmly up to the front door where he proceeded to unlock it with a key out of his pocket.

Kat cautiously walked behind Ben, her eyes growing wide with pleasure at each of the rooms they entered.

'Ben! Whose house is this?'

'Do you like it?'

'It's beautiful, but whose is it?'

'It's yours. I told you I want to do something for us—this is our new home, all in your name, it's yours!'

He saw the tears that bulged her eyes, then rolled down her face and he moved quickly to wipe them away with his thumbs, cradling her cheeks between his hands.

'Tell me they're tears of happiness.'

'Oh, Ben.'

'What?' His hands moved to her shoulders, massaging in a circular motion.

'It's the kindest, most generous thing anyone has ever done for me. But what does it mean? Are we going to live together?'

His hands slowed, and she seized his eyes and would not let them go.

'We'll work something out.'

'What? You're always saying that—work something out, but what? Are you working out how to leave your wife? Or me?'

Her watery eyes still held him and for the first time in his relationship with Kat, her eyes were transparent and plain to read.

'The truth. I've been avoiding it and I know that's not what you want to hear. The children, India and Kenya, you know how I love my kids. I can't walk away from them. They're so young... I worry what life will become without me being there daily.'

Her eyes lowered and released him as she turned away, but he gently pulled her back by the chin, forcing her to look at him.

'I love you. I'll live between London and Jamaica; I'll find a way to make something work.' He was desperate and hoped she would understand his position. 'But I can't leave my kids now.'

She moved from the circle of his arms and walked over by the window looking onto the green back lawn with the sea in the distance. 'I don't expect you to. You had nothing to do with my choice, but everything to do with my dream. I have only myself to blame. You were destined to come and you came. And as a result of that I got what Mother Cynthy predicted; she told me you'd be a man with secrets, and you were.' She moved from the window to sink herself into the soft leather chair. He watched confused as she rubbed her back against the chair, enjoyment distracting her for a brief moment. 'I may have done you wrong, Ben.' She looked directly into his eyes.

'I doubt it.' He kneeled beside the chair and kissed her lips.

'It may not be what you want, but it was fate, Mother

Cynthy predicted it.'

He stroked her cheek, running his finger along her lips. 'I ached for you, Kat. All those months away... I could only dream of touching you.'

'I need you to listen to me now because I may not have the courage to tell you another time. Please.'

He frowned. 'Okay. Is it bad news?'

'Not to me.'

'Not to you, but it could be to me?

Her silence made him anxious.

'What is it, Kat? Is there someone else you want to tell me about?'

She nodded cautiously.

'Is it another man?' Just saying the words wrenched his gut. He leaned away from her.

'Ben, I–I–I—'

'Don't beat about the bush, Kat,' his voice was sharp, 'just let me have it.'

'Well, he's not quite a man yet, but he is my little man,' she laughed nervously.

Ben could not believe she could make a joke out of this. Perhaps he hadn't been plain enough in his feelings for her. She hadn't taken him serious.

'The other love in my life, apart from you is Shadrach Thornton Benjamin Lewis. We call him Shaddy.' She exhaled. 'He's six months old and he's your son.'

Thirty-five

Kat

It seemed an age before he moved and until he did Kat dared not breathe. She watched emotions flash across his face. Disbelief, then amazement, replaced by scepticism, then dismay.

'What did you say?' His voice was barely a whisper.

'We have a son, Shaddy and he's six months old.'

'What are you saying?' He was clearly puzzled.

'We have a son,' Kat repeated, anxious.

'How?' he couldn't help but ask, even if he knew it was a ridiculous question.

'Ben—'

He stood to his feet and paced the room and Kat could see the numbness claiming him.

'My head is reeling but I can't find the questions. You have a baby, my baby, a son! How... I'm...'

'Don't look at me like that, Ben, please.'

He stood frozen in helplessness, his hands hanging loosely by his side, his shoulders drooped and the darkness that entered his eyes filled them with a sadness that was too painful for her to see.

'I know you must want answers... and I must give

them to you.'

He made no move to speak.

'I found out I was pregnant soon after you left. I wasn't surprised, Mother Cynthy saw me swimming with fishes, she predicted it. I told you this. To start, I secretly wanted a baby. I thought by having a baby I would have everything I needed. My life has been empty, Ben, I never realised how much until I met you. But when you said you were married, I tried to distance my feelings, you know I did. I didn't want to love a married man— but I so wanted you to be the man from across the sea, the one Mother Cynthy said would make a baby with me. I fought every serious thought about us, especially after you told me about your marriage, but you were... are so irresistible, I couldn't help myself. I wanted you... I want you and I love you.'

She couldn't stand the way he was looking at her as though she was a stranger speaking a foreign language. It had all gone so wrong and now she was drowning, with no branch to hold on to. Mother Cynthy hadn't warned her about this.

'Ben, say something! Cuss me if you must! Do something... just stop looking at me like I've just ripped out your heart.'

Her outburst was met with further silence as his pain-coloured eyes moved over her. What on earth had happened? What was he hearing?

'Ben... please, talk.'

She could no longer take the silence, the pain that poured from him.

'I don't blame you if you hate me. Miss Ruthie, my friends Rosie and Paula and even Columbus said you had a right to know about your son. I should have told you before now, I'm sorry.'

She walked to the door. His eyes followed but he made no attempt to stop her. It broke her heart.

*

The solo bark of Eden, Mother Cynthy's Labrador welcomed Kat as she made her way up the steep path and waded through the riotous plants that ran around the purple house. Two bleached white grave stones stood like guards on the right hand side of the front lawn, the final resting place for Mother Cynthy's parents, both dead within weeks of each other over thirty years ago. The friendly dog chased his tail, circling Kat, clearly excited. She would on normal occasions give into a two-minute romp with the animal, but today the weight she carried made her shoo him away. She walked around the back to find Mother Cynthy picking herbs and stacking them in the basket beside her on the ground. The strong, mixed herbal scents from the plants and bushes created a healing and calming environment and Kat was briefly pulled back into her childhood.

Cynthy spoke without turning around, 'I dropped a knife and fork and it made a cross, so I was expecting a visitor with a gripe. Then about ten minutes ago Eden started chase his tail like a mad dawg and I know I would see you.' She finally turned to face Kat. 'Why your face looking like thunder? Come sit down and let it all out.' She led her to the front of the house to sit on the veranda.

Kat sat sulkily on the cushioned straw chair, folding her arms across her chest and looking miserably at the old woman.

'Life simple but it isn't easy, huh?'

She nodded dejectedly. 'You saw fishes in my palms, you saw the man to make a baby with me... you knew he had secrets... what else? Before Shaddy was born I dreamt a fish suffocating in a pond, should I be worried?'

'Such a dream would signal a loss, a miscarriage, not necessarily you, but someone connected to you... that was not your fate.'

Kat's mood did not change. 'What more can you tell me?'

'I tell you all I see.'

'You didn't tell me I would love him and that it would feel like this.'

'I can only tell you what I see. I told you there would always be a lot more I can't see. What you expect? Plain sailing, is that what you after?'

The old woman's words rendered Kat speechless. She had known the score, the outcome of loving a married man. If only she could turn the clock back. She wouldn't undo everything; just unpick the moment when it all changed, when love took root. She could pin point the exact moments, feel that turbulent and uncontrollable passion engulfing her like a tidal wave the first time he stripped her naked and looked at her with such longings. The moment his parted lips met hers. The moments spent laughing, looking into the skies, eating, feeding each other, reading, and talking. If she could only go back and manipulate those moments so they meant nothing. If only.

'What shall I do?'

'Let me see your palms.' She pulled Kat's hand into her own. 'There's a storm to come but it clears... and the twist in this line,' her chubby finger travelled along a line that faded, 'it mean a visit from a stranger.' She frowned.

'What do you see, Mother Cynthy, tell me.'

'It's a stranger with a heavy shadow.'

'What does it mean?'

'Not sure but you'll know soon enough.'

If Ben still wanted her she would have to call on her innermost strength in order to demand of him that he make a choice. Yes, she must. He must choose between his wife and her, Shadrach and his daughters. It was the only way.

It was late afternoon when Kat left Mother Cynthy, feeling like a stuffed bag of stones had replaced her gut. She took a stroll down to the beach and stopped off at Rosie's Shack. Not many people were there. Nellie Potato's grandson, Dwayne, who had another tourist, this time a brunette with sea blue eyes who looked far too sensible to fall for someone like Dwayne, who after all was just a gigolo. He was doing well. He had his own glass-bottom boat, rumours said bought by the "fat white lady" he had before this one, and he had started building a house for his wife and their three children, such was the generosity of these foreign women with big purses.

Rosie led Kat to the back of the shack where her three roomed board house was situated. The small yard was clean and organised with a variety of flowers planted in old car tires painted white and strategically placed around the house for enhancement. A line led from the zinc roof to a branch of a breadfruit tree where clothes hung drying in the hot sun. A thin dog lay sleeping on its side under the makeshift shelter of an old car roof, propped up by four wooden poles. There was no veranda but three white plastic chairs and a table by the front door was host to guests and families. They sat around the table and Rosie passed a bottle of water to Kat, keeping an eye on her pot of chicken soup bubbling and steaming on the wooden fire in the yard, which she would sell later to her regular customers.

'Candy Eyes is here?'

Kat nodded, undoing the bottle and gulping down the cold liquid.

'You look beat down.'

Kat shrugged her shoulders. 'I'm okay. Your soup smells delicious.'

Rosie licked her lips. 'Thanks. Sorry to upset you the other day, but you know I always speak my mind.'

'Don't apologise. You have the right to an opinion.'

'I keep my big mouth shut, I don't tell a soul... first secret I ever keep in my life for longer than two days!'

A shadow of a smile touched Kat's lips. 'Thanks.'

'So,' Rosie said watching her closely, 'you tell him about Shaddy?'

'Yes. He's speechless. I think he's mad with me. I left and he didn't call me back.'

'The man's in shock, girl. You live on another planet if you really believed everything would be happy-ever-after. You know what you going to do? Realistically?'

'I know only one thing, Rosie. I want Ben. But to have him will hurt people he loves. That's difficult, but I have to think about myself and Shaddy, why shouldn't I?'

Rosie shook her head. 'All that education—'

'Education doesn't make you immune to mistakes,

Rosie, I made a mistake!' said Kat, frustrated with her friend's comments.

Rosie shook her head again. 'Eh-eh, in the beginning yes,' she pointed a wagging finger, 'but now you've made a decision.'

'You're really mad at me,' Kat told her.

'Not mad,' Rosie said wearily, 'just sad, you know. How will good ever come of this? You think about his wife and how she love him? And his pickney? You really think about this, Kat?'

Kat wanted to hear Rosie tell her she was right, not to think about Ben's wife. She wanted understanding about her relationship with Ben and encouragement to fight for him. The fact that she was feeling so distraught about her decision to make him choose only served to frustrate her more. She began crying and Rosie pulled her close, comforting her.

'If it make you feel this bad you have to let it go, Kat,' Rosie urged gently. 'Just let it go.'

Thirty-six
Ben
Jamaica

Sunset had come and gone as Ben sat with Shadrach on his lap around Miss Ruthie's dining table, a drink standing in Miss Ruthie's very best crystal glass before him waiting to see Kat, since her revelation. She came to an abrupt halt on entering the house. Her eyes were transparent. He could see she was in torment and he wanted to make it better as quickly as possible. He brushed his cheek against Shadrach's soft curls and smiled directly at her.

'There you are, we been waiting for you. Shaddy's daddy had to introduce himself, where you been all this time?' Miss Ruthie challenged.

Kat's eyes swelled with tears and she made a rush for her room. Miss Ruthie looked apologetically at Ben. 'I'll go see what gripe her.'

Ben quickly handed Miss Ruthie the baby. 'If you don't mind I'd like to talk to her.'

'You think you can manage her?' Miss Ruthie asked with obvious doubt. 'Her head and ears are hard and she slow to take advice.'

Ben smiled. 'I know.'

The room was small and sparsely furnished. A single bed, a chest of drawers with a small television on top, a handmade cot and a time-worn arm chair whose threads were thin and faded. The floral curtains matched the bedspread and there had been a great attempt at making it comfortable. The baby blue coloured walls were adorned by her pencil sketches and a picture of a black Christ with his hand crossed over his heart hung above her bed.

Under his feet was highly polished red tile floor and he suddenly felt he should remove his shoes; it might leave prints on such a shine. She sat on the bed with arms hugging her knees, that neutral look occupying her eyes again.

'Hey, sweet girl,' he greeted while kicking off his shoes.

'It's a gift.'

He looked puzzled. 'Huh?'

'The picture of Christ over my bed. It belonged to Old Man but he gave it to me. He's coming out of the hospital in a few weeks and he'll be living here with us.'

'That's nice.'

'He's a wonderful soul.'

Ben took the few steps to stand by her bed. 'May I sit on your bed?'

'Silly question.'

'I'm taking no chances with you, lady, you'd most probably tell me about some law of nature that was compromised by my sitting on your bed without permission.'

Kat gave way to a weak smile.

'That's a start.' He hesitated. 'Kat, why didn't you tell me?' It was the burning question, the first of thousands he wanted answers to.

'The truth is it was my dream, not yours so it's hard to explain.'

'But to go through nine months of pregnancy, then a labour followed by another six months of nursing a baby, all without my knowledge—me, the father... I'm just baffled as to why you would do such a thing.'

She rested her chin on her knees and stared ahead miserably. 'I got it all wrong and I've messed up.'

He saw the tears gather in her eyes and reached for her but she resisted, flapping her hands in front of her frantically as though she was warding off a bee attack.

'Miss Ruthie told me you could have died giving birth to Shaddy. She said you shouldn't have put your life at such great risk, and I agree with her.' He saw anger flash in her eyes. 'I know you had your reasons but you were wrong. When I think back to the first time I returned to Jamaica after our meeting, you were four months pregnant and I didn't know. You could have told me then, Kat.'

'And now that I have, what will you do?'

Ben heaved a heavy sigh. 'I need to understand this. You've given me a lot to think about in the last couple of hours and there's so much to take on board. I've just discovered I have a son, a baby boy! Do you have any idea what this means to me?'

He knew she didn't. He hadn't told her about his deep desire to have a son or that Claire's ectopic had put an end to that dream. Now suddenly it wasn't a dream, it was real and he had a son.

'I believed totally in Mother Cynthy's prediction and it came through. I wanted a baby more than anything at the time but I just didn't dream this far ahead, after the baby... I didn't know I'd fall for a married man, which has made it so difficult.'

Pangs of guilt rippled throughout him. 'We didn't plan our feelings for each other. Do you wish you'd never met me?' he asked pensively.

'No, no, no!' She shook her head furiously. 'Don't think like that. It was destined to be you. Mother Cynthy predicted that I would make a baby with a man from across the sea. Then she saw me swimming with fishes just a day before I met you. The day I met you—I knew you were the one.'

She could still amaze him with her unwavering belief in the unbelievable. Mother Cynthy and her predictions. The river taking from you if you don't bring it a gift. The reasons he loved her intensified with each meeting, and he could not stay angry. A son meant he now had a dynasty bearing his name. This new feeling was exciting. He had a son. He could hardly believe it.

'I can't say I understand this any more than I did when you first told me, all I know is that I have a son.'

'Things can't return to how they were, Ben. You need to make some decisions. I can't live like this anymore, I just can't.'

It was Shadrach's crying that brought their conversation to an end.

'He wants a bottle.' She stood. 'I hope Miss Ruthie heard nothing.'

'Can I feed him?' Ben offered.

'Sure.'

Miss Ruthie was sat on the veranda in her rocking chair with Shadrach on her lap, his head resting against her breast as she tried to hush his cries.

She looked up quizzically as Ben and Kat appeared.

'I think his teeth bothering him; no bottle can comfort him right now,' she told them.

Ben lifted his small son into his arms, still amazed by his existence. The baby cooed and smiled up at him causing a stream of emotion to erupt. He looked so much like Kenya when she was a baby, the eyes and little button nose and of course a fine line of side burns which vanished by his ear lobes. He inhaled the baby smell of his son and reality seeped in with it. Claire-Louise. This would devastate her. Then there were the children, India and Kenya to consider. Two worlds were fighting for dominance. He felt all control leave him.

Kat was right; they shared a destiny and now had a child that bound their lives together. She was also correct in that decisions had to be made, but he didn't know how.

Thirty-seven

Kat

Kat wiped her eyes on the pillow for the umpteenth time only to have fresh tears spring up again. She lay on her back squeezing them together tightly in order to prevent the stream but they forced themselves out the sides of her eyes until she felt the trickle in her ears. The night sky had been replaced by dawn and she could hear Miss Ruthie's movements as the old lady prepared the shop for the day ahead. The thought flickered quickly across her mind that she should get up to assist with setting out the provisions, but the rocks of despair still bound her stomach. Ben had returned to the guest house last night without asking her to come with him. Not that she would have, but to have been asked might have given reprieve to the anguish.

'You sleeping, child?' Miss Ruthie entered the room, walking over to sit on the side of her bed. Kat moved her legs to make more room.

'No, just resting.'

She peeped into the cot at her sleeping grandson. 'He really looks like his daddy, huh? Spitting image.'

Kat did not respond.

'You been crying, child?

Kat shook her head in denial, fully aware that Miss Ruthie knew different.

'All in all I think Ben took the news of having a son him never know about very well. Some men would just walk away with no conscience. You very lucky to have a young man like that. Don't make time run out... learn from me,' she said with real sadness that told Kat she was thinking about Old Man.

Miss Ruthie's voice floated from a distance as Kat's mind wondered back to her predicament. Who would Ben choose? She felt the tears close again and quickly blinked them back, thankful that it went unnoticed by her mother.

'I was wrong 'bout him. I always think foreign men only out to use and abuse but him seem different... full of manners,' she broke off to chuckle, 'and very charming. I can see marriage is on the card. Shaddy need him daddy. You have to explain to Columbus—'

'There'll be no marriage, Miss Ruthie.'

'You joking, right?'

'No.'

Kat held the hard and steady gaze of her mother, knowing she would have to arm herself for battle.

'You breaking sticks at your ears again. What is wrong with you? Why at every turn you have to fight me? The opportunity to marry the father of your child presents itself and you saying it's not what you want? You not understanding how I delay, delay with Old Man.' Miss Ruthie was clearly distressed.

'It's complicated.'

'It's complicated,' Miss Ruthie responded sarcastically.

She threw her hands in the air as she faced Kat, her eyes hard with anger and frustration. 'What is wrong with you? Why if I say A you must say B and if I say B you choose C? Your father turning in him grave right now at the foolishness his educated child has become.'

Kat shrugged her shoulders and looked towards the window. A stream of sun had broken the dark morning sky and had tunnelled its light through a gap in the curtain to land on Shadrach's sleeping face.

'Miss Ruthie,' Kat spoke with caution. 'I can't marry Ben right now. Can you just leave well alone, it's my life and I can make decisions for me and Shaddy.'

'Why?' Miss Ruthie demanded. 'Why you can't marry him now? If you can spread your legs for a man, carry his child, why you won't marry him?'

Shadrach stirred and Kat leaned over his cot and patted his back. It was also an opportunity to gather her thoughts and avoid Miss Ruthie's persistent questioning.

'Ben bought me a house... a three-bedroom in Meadow View,' her voice took on springs as she tried to lighten the mood. 'It has hot water, a big kitchen and front and back lawn. It would be good for us to move there for when Old Man comes out of hospital.'

'Him buy you a house? In Meadow View?'

Kat nodded, her face breaking into a smile.

'Him buy you a house and you refuse to marry him?' Miss Ruthie's face took on horrified. 'I really don't think the fancy education your father paid for has done you a scrap of good. It is a good thing he's not here to see this.' She gave Kat the elevator look, up then down before walking out shaking her head and talking to herself.

Kat arrived at the guest house while the night staff was still on duty, Shadrach wrapped tightly in a blue blanket cradled in her arms. She made her way down the corridor to his room, responding to the polite 'good mornings' of the staff. Outside his door she knocked lightly. He opened the door in his boxer shorts.

'Hey, sweet girl.' He placed a kiss on her cheek and held out his arms to take Shadrach. 'I was wondering if you were real, or if I'd just dreamt you,' he told the sleeping baby.

She followed him into the room and watched in silence as he placed the baby on the bed, positioning pillows around him. He turned to her. 'Let's sit on the balcony and enjoy some of that morning sun.'

Ben sat on one of the straw chairs and she stood with her back to the balcony railings. His eyes flickered with tiredness and uncertainty. 'You okay?'

'You haven't slept, have you?' She was concerned.

He shook his head in agreement, running a hand over his braids. 'You've given me a whole lot to think about.'

It was then it really all came clear to her, what she had really done to him, to his life, to herself and her baby.

'I think we both know that it's too much and very unfair of you to expect me and Shaddy to contend with seeing you a few times a year. We need security, normality, you understand?'

She saw the devastation in his eyes, the welled-up tears that were blinked away by rapid movements, the teeth that bit his bottom lips nervously and she longed to move into the arms she knew offered love so deep, so sweet that nothing else mattered. He was looking at her now with a mixture of pain and want and she knew she could not resist him.

'I somehow fooled myself into thinking I could make this all work out.' He rubbed his chin and she heard the sand paper sound caused by unshaven skin. 'I love you, Kat. I fell and I fell hard for you, and if it wasn't for my–my girls and Claire, things would be different. I feel I've let you down... I hate what I've—'

'No, no. It's me who's let you down. I didn't think beyond the moment. I guess we both didn't.'

'A son. I can still hardly believe it... and now you want me to make a choice. I hope you know it's the hardest thing I've ever been asked in my life. I'm not sure I can.'

'You must,' she urged softly.

'Suppose I choose you?' He stood in front of her, close to her as she looked up at him.

He stroked her face with two fingers, circling her lips. 'Nothing makes sense without you—' his voice broke.

'You go home, Ben. Go home and talk to your family, make your decision and don't call me until you do.'

'That would be impossible.'

She fell against him and his arms found her and pulled her close as his lips sought hers. They kissed for a long moment before he led her inside and she couldn't help wondering if this would be the last time they shared a bed.

Thirty-eight
Kat

The waves rushed to her feet like an obedient dog excited by its mistress as she stood on the shore looking out to sea. She wondered what it would be like to venture that far out into the vast ocean, just as a plane flew overhead making the sound of roaring thunder and leaving behind a white trail across the sky. Ben was the other side of that sea, had been for the past three weeks, beyond the sky further than her eyes could see. It was never supposed to be like this. She ran to the shelter of her throne, under the palm trees. She reached for her bag and pulled out her sketch pad and pencil, then began to write as though a spirit had taken control of her hand.

> *Ben,*
> *Choose me.*
> *All my love—Kat*

She left the beach after sunset and walked towards a waiting taxi, the letter crunched up in her pocket. She had no intention of sending it. It was simply a way of releasing the mounting torrent of distress that had accompanied her since he went back to London.

'Kat!'

She turned to see Rosie struggling with two boxes of spring water. Kat waved the taxi on and assisted her friend to carry them to her shack on the beach. After packing the bottles into the fridge, Rosie invited her to sit.

'You doing okay?'

Kat looked towards the sea. It was still. 'I'm in limbo, Rosie. I told Ben to go home and make his choice. He's supposed to call me when he does. I'm just waiting. I feel I can't move on until I hear from him.'

'Waiting? Why? You need to start living your life. Candy Eyes is living his with wifey. Why don't you move in your new house? A change might make you feel better.'

Kat considered this. Moving to Meadow View would give her a break. But to leave Miss Ruthie and Old Man, she wasn't sure she could.

'I would worry too much about Miss Ruthie and Old Man. She won't move out of her house, not for one day.'

'It's a break, Kat,' Rosie encouraged. 'You can still visit Miss Rootie everyday.'

Kat admitted it was a good idea. A complete change might help to keep her mind off Ben. It wouldn't be permanent, she told herself.

*

'It look like a dry storm coming,' Miss Ruthie stated as she walked around her house, closing all the windows. 'Let's hope it pass and tomorrow bring calm. No sense in setting out the provisions and it better Young Tin-Tin keep Charmaine tied up in the hills.'

Tin-Tin, their neighbour's grandson had taken over looking after Charmaine since Old Man's stroke. His absence was taking some getting use to because no matter what, Kat always expected him to come through the gate each morning and she knew Miss Ruthie did too. He had progressed and could walk with the aid of a stick. His speech was slightly slurred but he was well enough and soon he would be coming home. Miss Ruthie bought a single bed for herself because she wanted to make sure Old Man would be comfortable in her bed, despite the fact they were not yet married and folks were already talking. She no longer cared. Her encounter with the real possibility of losing him had given her senses a good shake and she knew, at the grand old age of 69 that what people thought didn't have to matter. However, she had already booked a date for the wedding, a private affair taking place in her front yard officiated by new, young, Pastor Jack who had livened up the church.

Kat was slowly packing hers and Shadrach's belongings, void of all the joy she thought would accompany this day. Ben had been gone for a month now.

Miss Ruthie watched with a solemn look on her face. 'So, you really going to move out?'

'Just for a break, Miss Ruthie.'

'I stop trying to make sense out of you ever since you sent Ben away. Mark my word you will live to regret that.'

'I already do,' she said simply.

Miss Ruthie pulled a chair from the dining table and

sat down, dipping her hand into the small brown paper bag and pulling out a hand full of uncooked rice.

'What really happen between you and Ben? I know you love him. I know that without a shadow a doubt and him seems to love you too, so what is it?' She filled her mouth with rice and began crunching. 'There's something you not telling me.'

'There's a whole lot I'm not telling you,' her tone was glum. 'Do one thing for me, Miss Ruthie, please.' Tears weighed heavy in her voice.

'Of course, child, anything.' Miss Ruthie leaned forward, concerned.

'Don't ask me anything more about Ben. It hurts too much.'

'It's a great pity—good men are hard to find.'

'I know.'

*

She had not anticipated such loneliness, living on her own with Shadrach in their new three-bedroom house in Meadow View, up in the hills where at nights she could look down over the valley and see the lights of some of the homes in the Meadows. It was so different from what she was used to. The neighbours all seemed to have fancy cars or jeeps and no time to converse with each other, just a royal wave as they climbed into their vehicles and went about their business. She had no idea of their professions, only that they all earned a great deal of money. No-one stopped by the gate to chat, not like at home with Miss Ruthie; and the houses were separated by high walls or gates and it wasn't clear if they were locking themselves in or people out. Rosie and Ras

Solomon passed by to see her and she was glad of their company. They were so impressed with her new home that an idea immediately sprang to her mind.

'Why don't you and the children live here, Rosie? It's too big for just Shaddy and me. Ras Solomon, you can come too.'

Rosie grinned and looked around the room eagerly. 'It's a pretty house, Kat, but I don't think I could afford to pay your rent.'

'But Rosie, you wouldn't have to pay me rent. You can live with me free of charge.' Kat knew she sounded desperate, and she was. Desperate and lonely. Having Rosie live with her would fill her time, her life.

'Well that don't make no sense! My children would wreck the place and I have no money to give you to fix it back. It's such a pretty house, but I need to live where people are real. I wouldn't fit in here, Kat and I would miss the beach.'

Kat was frantic to change Rosie's mind. 'Nonsense.' She took hold of Rosie's hands, squeezing them. 'You need a chance like this, for your children to wake up to running water… hot water to bathe in, and a flush toilet. Give it a try, please.'

Rosie looked solemnly at her friend. 'Me living with you is not what you really need, it won't solve nutting,' she said meaningfully.

Ras Solomon had his say as well: 'I couldn't live in a place like this, with all them spiritless people around with them big car and expensive clothes living behind high gates and walls, like a prison. No, I feel safer in mi little house in de hills. But thank you for thinking of us.'

Only nine days had passed before she decided to pack their belongings and return to familiarity, ready for Miss Ruthie's 'I told you so' look, but she would welcome it.

Miss Ruthie of course was happy to see them back with unashamed opened arms and lots of 'I told you so's.'

'I miss all the noise you and Shaddy make around the house.' She smiled, hugging Shadrach to her bosom. 'A big house is nice, but only if it full with life and family and companionship. It has been good having Old Man, he's himself again. Old Man, Kat and Shaddy are back.'

It seemed to take an age before Old Man's face appeared in the living room. Miss Ruthie immediately rushed to aid his sitting on the sofa. 'Miss Rootie, I know how to sit,' his grin was lopsided when he smiled at Kat and she hugged him warmly.

'What you going to do 'bout the house? You selling it?'

She shook her head vigorously. 'No, it's for Shadrach. I'll rent it for now and when he's old enough, he can decide.'

'You need a husband, Kat. Don't be stubborn about love like I was. Now all I have to live with is regret. I regret I never marry Old Man before now.'

Of course Miss Ruthie did not know the whole story—that Ben was already married—and Kat had no intention of telling her. It was her burden to bear and bear it she would.

Columbus returned in mid-October, winter season in the Meadows where the breeze was cooler during the days and carried a hint of chill in the evenings. Although the tourists still talked of the searing heat and went around sleeveless, the natives donned cardigans and jackets and younger children wore woollen hats and were wrapped in sheets or blankets by their parents.

Columbus came laden with gifts, more so than ever before and his long unruly hair had been cropped to his shoulders in an orderly way she had never seen before. Gone were the worn and tattered trousers and the stretched out T-shirts. Instead he donned khaki-coloured chinos and a green and beige checked shirt. The transformation was one from a 1960s hippy to a 21st century school teacher.

'My God, Kat, he's grown so big... and he's crawling already,' Columbus enthused on entering the house.

'He won't stop trying.' She smiled, genuinely happy to see her friend.

'So do I get a hug or what?' he asked.

She threw herself into his outstretched arms and held on as if her life depended on it. He laughed, surprised at the new passion in which he was greeted.

'Your hair? Why?' She sounded disappointed.

'I wanted a change. Where's Miss Ruthie?'

'Gone with Old Man to Bible study. He seems to enjoy it too. They got married by the new Pastor Jack a week after he came home. His speech is pretty good, though he doesn't walk as fast as before, but it's early days yet. Miss Ruthie is doing her very best to turn him into a Christian.'

'I heard. But Old Man will not be a good Christian. It is him who taught me to drink rum without getting drunk.'

Kat looked surprised. 'And how do you do that?'

'The trick is to fill your stomach with much food and after every mouthful of rum, you drink two mouthfuls of water. '

She laughed. 'Oh Col, I'm so happy to see you, and you haven't spoken a word of French yet.'

He grinned. 'I was trying to impress you, no more need for that but I think I should go home to Paris more often if it means I'm going to be greeted like this all the time. What do you say, little one?' He bent down to pick up Shadrach, who whined and wriggled in his arms until Columbus had to put him down.

'He's forgotten me,' Columbus's voice was filled with disappointment.

Kat picked up her son and hugged him. 'He's just fussy like his daddy.' She bit into her lips as soon as she realised what she had said. It was too late, Columbus looked crestfallen and there was nothing she could do about that.

The Meadows prepared for Harvest, a Christian celebration that brought the town folks out in numbers in their best dress. The colourful lights flashed around the entrance of the church, creating nearly as much excitement as Christmas for the children.

Kat was taking part by organising for her and Shadrach to join the annual trek from the Meadows up to Meadow Height, which Miss Ruthie strongly disapproved of. Walking five miles up into the breezy hills in the mid of winter had never harmed anyone before, but no-one in the little town suffered with sickle cell the way her daughter did. The look on her face said it all, 'There you go again, thinking you're superwoman.'

Kat continued wrapping fried fish and cutting hard dough bread to fill the picnic breakfast basket. The skies showed signs of daybreak and the cocks crows echoed as they drifted across the Meadows.

'I think it very unwise to take you and the young baby up in that breezy hills; make sure you both wrap up against the breeze,' she warned with a point of her wagging finger.

'Let me be like everyone else and enjoy Harvest. For once just give me an easy time, Miss Ruthie.'

'No reason why you can't come with me and Old Man in the church van. We can wait for everyone to come down from the hills.'

Kat closed the basket having put all she wanted in. There was a great deal of food but that was how things were done in the Meadows. Everyone would bring food and it would be shared out among the masses once they returned from the hills and settled on the town's vast green.

'Miss Ruthie, I feel strong enough to make the walk. I promise no swimming in the river,' she teased, 'but I want to make that walk with my son. Columbus will carry him.'

'You always doing what you want, nobody don't matter but you. From you born I been pleading with you to see sense but your head is as hard as nails. You get yourself pregnant for a foreigner who didn't even know 'bout his child and you think it alright.'

Her mother's anger over her pregnancy had not diminished over the year.

'I did something you said I never could. I didn't commit a crime. I did what normal women do, Miss

298

Ruthie, you above all should understand. Look how you wanted a baby and that baby came out sick, keeping you in and out of hospital for years. Despite all of that, would you change it all if you could? Would you rather I was never born?'

Miss Ruthie had no answer.

'Aren't you proud of me, Miss Ruthie?' Kat beamed at her mother hoping to lighten the mood.

'Yes, I'm proud, Kat. But I fear for you too. You still don't seem to know your danger. You're still like that wild, stubborn little girl who want to do what everyone else does, not realising she can't.'

'But I can. I always could. It was your belief in what happened to Aunt Doris that caused so much fear, and for nothing.'

It was Mama Gem, Pa Gem, Old Man and a solemn Miss Ruthie who dropped Kat, Columbus and Shadrach in the town centre where they joined the large group who would be making the trek up to Meadow Heights.

'See you soon.' Pa Gem smiled but Miss Ruthie kept her head straight as the truck drove slowly away.

Kat and Columbus lingered towards the end of the crowd, taking their time to stroll and observe the various cedar and almond trees that was indigenous to the area.

The group soon split into two, as the fitter and faster walkers took the lead, leaving mostly the parents with young children and the elders behind. Out of tune hymns rang loud but no-one cared. Halfway through the trek Kat admitted to herself that Miss Ruthie may have been right. The walk was uphill most of the way and she began to feel weary. Columbus was quick to notice the slower pace she adopted and offered to carry her on his back and let Rosie carry Shadrach. She refused with a smile. 'I'll be alright, this pace is good,' she told him.

The pre-dawn skies had now given way to daybreak and the rising sun slowly took the chill out of the breeze. On their arrival at the top of the hill, Kat sat on a log at the side of the dirt path, thankful for the relief it gave her aching back. The crowds continued singing and the church van carrying Old Man, Miss Ruthie and the Gems among others had parked at the side of the narrow dirt road.

'Is anybody sitting there?' The unfamiliar English tone caused her to look up into a pair of kind-worn grey eyes. They belonged to a middle-aged white man, a gentleman by sight. He removed his Panama hat; his thick grey hair covered only the sides of his head, leaving the middle bald and tanned. He wore a colourful shirt, plain white shorts, socks with sandals and carried a knapsack. 'May I?' he asked graciously.

'Yes, fine.' She smiled and shifted to accommodate him.

A comfortable silence fell between them.

'You're new to the Meadows,' she told him, eyeing him curiously.

His laugh was typically English.

'Yes, it's my first time here, my name's Henry. I've heard a lot about it from my daughter. I came to see for myself why she was so impressed with the place, enough to want to give up everything to live here. It is very beautiful, what I've seen so far.' He sounded like a voice on the BBC World Service.

She became intrigued. 'You mean she's leaving

England to live here, in the Meadows?'

He nodded, a little weary. 'Yes'.

'Are you worried about her?' Kat asked a touch timid, not knowing if she was being too nosey.

'It's for the love of a good man,' he said dryly, his eyes cast in front of him looking out, straight ahead.

He continued, 'I suppose love is love, isn't it? My daughter tells me we don't choose who we fall in love with, but I have to disagree. And Jamaica is so far away from Cambridge. I'm not sure she is seeing things clearly right now.'

Kat felt a pang of empathy for the man. He seemed so kind, so warm and to be really suffering with the situation he had been dealt. He smiled at Kat, only a hint of embarrassment in his eyes. 'Perhaps I've said too much,' he said.

She was struggling inside trying hard to not put herself in the picture, but once she'd had the thought it became relentless in her mind and she suddenly blurted out, 'Why shouldn't your daughter be with her love?'

The answer came with a deep sigh. 'I mean, he seems to be a nice enough young man,' he frowned slightly.

'But you feel there's something... not right about him?'

He scratched his beard. 'To be honest, I've only seen him when he comes to the hotel to see us. I've not met his family yet, not sure why. My daughter has met his grandmother and sings her praises. I'm sure I'll meet them before I leave. My wife would never forgive me if I were to go back home without those kind of details... she's very family-orientated, you know.'

'You want some advice?'

He chortled, briefly covering his mouth. 'I think you've been very free with it so far.'

Kat blushed. 'I don't believe in coincidences, so I think you and I met for a reason,' she announced with humour. 'I think I'm supposed to make true love happen for your daughter and her beau.'

He tilted forward with laughter. 'How will you do that?'

'By suggesting you allow her beau to visit you all in... Cambridge, is it? Then you'll get to know him and he will get to know you better and also experience a different part of the world.'

'In the end, my wife and I just want our daughter happy.' Again the deep-belly sigh. 'She's had it rather tough, miscarriages, divorce, battled depression and won. She's emotionally fragile so if this is what it takes,' he shrugged his shoulders.

Kat swallowed a deep sense of sadness for the girl and her father. She believed in love especially because of her situation and felt an overwhelming desire to make this man and his daughter happy.

'I wonder if I know him?'

'His name is Dwayne.'

Kat became serious, dread pooling in her stomach. 'And what is his grandmother's name?'

He looked confused at her changed manner. 'A rather odd one. Miss Nellie, or Nellie Potato, my daughter says she's called.'

Kat struggled to contain her anger.

'You were right to have doubts; your feelings about him are correct... Dwayne is a married man. He has three kids; Dwayne Jr, Donovan and Letesha.'

Henry looked bereft. 'My God! Are you sure? This can't be... My God, oh my God... She might not believe—'

Caught between anger at Dwayne and sadness for this man and his daughter, Kat interrupted, 'I can give you the address and directions to his house, take your daughter on Sunday afternoon, you'll find him at home with his wife and children, having dinner, it's routine in the Meadows. No matter who you are or where you go in the week, on Sundays you find your family.'

'I must be old here at seventy-one, and out of touch with modern things. What could possess a man to leave his wife and three children, for–for two weeks of summer romance? It's ridiculous. Why treat a woman who loves you like this? That goes for his wife too, because he's been lying to her and she'll be hurt by this. Selfish bastard. Theresa is so fragile, you understand? Oh my God, I don't know how she'll take this.'

Kat forced herself to breathe steadily. 'It'll hurt her now, but she'll be better off without him in the long run. Like you said, what a way to treat someone who loves you. He's been playing with two lives, more including his kids. What a way to treat someone who loves you,' she repeated.

Henry stood up and she joined him, tears swimming someplace far off because she just couldn't afford to cry now, at the reality that was trying to take shape in her head.

'I see why you don't believe in coincidences, maybe I won't now... if I hadn't met you today...' His voice trailed away, likely anticipating the emotional mountain he and his family were about to climb.

She nodded, 'I'm so sorry.'

'No. Thank you.'

He stood to his feet and held out a hand to assist her up. She wished him well and went to get on the bus back to town. Not noticing her demeanour as she made her way to their seats, Columbus chatted excitedly about what a great day it had been, leaving her to her thoughts about life and love and how talking to Henry felt something like divine intervention.

The following morning Kat slept through nature's natural alarms, the cock whose crow would stir her, Samson's bark, the pecks of the chickens, not to mention Miss Ruthie's noise.

'Quick Kat, get up, Shaddy sick, he having trouble breathing, quick, Kat,' urged Miss Ruthie, shaking her daughter.

Kat jumped up, wide awake in an instant, and rushed after Miss Ruthie, the cries leaving her mouth sounding foreign and not human as she reached for her baby.

'Phone Columbus and tell him to get here,' Miss Ruthie barked at Kat, feverishly tapping Shadrach's back. 'Let's get this baby straight to the hospital.'

*

The doctors were talking in hushed tones at the hospital as Kat and Columbus sat by Shadrach's cot. He was hooked up to machines and had wires coming out of him; a familiar sight which she had prayed would never befall her child.

His little chest rose up and down evenly and she was relieved to see there was no struggle to breathe. She bent down and kissed his cheek lightly and whispered, 'You're okay, baby boy, you're going to be fine.'

Miss Ruthie came later that evening. Kat met her with a relieved smile.

'He's going to be alright, Miss Ruthie, it's pneumonia but they have it under control.'

'Good. I phone his daddy and leave a message with the woman who picked up the phone. I tell her to make sure she informs Ben that his son sick in hospital.'

Kat viewed her mother with increasing despair, her eyes opening with the horror of what she was hearing. 'What woman? Where did you phone? Who gave you Ben's number?'

'He did, when he came. He say he live with his aunt so I leave the message with her... though she never sound happy about my call. She was very quiet while I explain 'bout Shaddy getting sick. She ask who I was and I tell her, she was very, very quiet.'

Every nerve in Kat's body became tense as she forced herself to sound normal. 'Who exactly did you tell her you were?'

Miss Ruthie looked strangely at her. 'The grandmother of Ben's son of course.'

Horror gripped Kat, tightening around her heart, seeping into her lungs making it difficult for her to breathe. She could not even find anger. Every emotion was suspended and she suddenly knew what it must feel like to see an express train heading for direct impact with you, and you are unable to move a muscle.

When she spoke it was a murmur, 'What have you done, Miss Ruthie, what have you done?'

Thirty-nine
Ben
London

Ben was an abandoned baby. He was ten years old when he realised what it actually meant and it threw his world into turmoil. He remembered the years of feeling rejected, the anger at a mother who could do such a thing, then the hopeless feeling of knowing there was nothing he could do to change it. That most of all sent him close to the edge. He felt like that now. Hopeless. He didn't want to hurt any of his two loves, leave them in hopelessness. He didn't want to reject Kat and he didn't want to abandon Claire. He knew that pain only too well.

The blood drained from his face and the room danced around him, flecks of flashing colours like a 70s disco. Ben sat quietly waiting for stillness. The guilt had escalated and it felt like too much, like he could not do another day being torn in two, spend another hour deceiving and tormenting the women he loved. Kat needed a decision. He needed to make it. He finally confided in his foster father.

Professor Faintheart sat facing him across his large

oak desk.

'I am disappointed in you, Ben, more than I can say. What on earth were you thinking? You've ruined many lives, not to mention your own. You had better forget about this nonsense,' the Professor spoke in a sharp whisper. 'I know you must take financial responsibility for your action, but for goodness' sake think about India, Kenya and your wife.'

Ben played absent-mindedly with his wedding band.

'If you love this woman,' the Professor warned, 'truly love her like you say, you will leave her alone, give her a chance to rebuild her life. You need to promise me you'll never see her again. Not to phone her. I'll do the communicating in terms of the child.'

Ben knew he could make no such promise. Eight weeks had staggered by since his return from Jamaica. He longed to call her but knew she would ask for the decision he didn't have. He was in limbo and knew something had to be done, he just didn't know what.

'I'm sorry, Prof; I have no excuses or explanations.' He closed his eyes for a long moment. 'I feel powerless over my feelings for her.'

'The heart has its reasons that reason does not know.' The Professor took off his glasses, and using the edge of his jumper cleaned them. 'You're going to have a lot of explaining to do to quite a few people, starting with your wife.'

Ben dropped his forehead into his hands in the hope of somehow gaining strength. 'I don't know how I let things go so far,' he confessed in a small voice. 'I don't know why I didn't walk away from her in the beginning, because now I feel I've let her down.'

'You've betrayed Claire-Louise and the girls.' He began pacing the office, his hands behind his back. 'I cannot believe you could be so mindless. Ben, at this moment in time, I despair for you.'

*

Ben left work early, much to the shock of his staff and headed straight for Bubs' small office in Notting Hill Gate. He had avoided telling his friend about his son because truth be known, he was still trying to get his head around the whole revelation. He signed in at the reception and the uniformed receptionist called through to let Bubs know he had a client. Ben made his way to the second floor, where a surprised Bubs stood waiting.

'What's wrong?' Bubs' wonder turned to concern.

Ben headed straight for the fridge, opening a can of Stella. Half of the tin's content was gone before he spoke.

'Listen carefully and don't say a word until I've finished,' Ben said with such seriousness that Bubs fell into quiet anticipation. 'Kat has had my son. She didn't tell me about him until I went out there in June—he's eight months now.'

The silence stretched. Bubs sat at his computer, a frown scarring his face.

'Bubs?' Ben enquired.

'Yeah, I hear ya. So she says she's had your son. How do you know it's yours? And what does she want— maintenance for the past eight months?' He chuckled.

'No, she doesn't want anything like that. He's mine alright, he's the image of Kenya.'

'Why didn't you tell me before now? You knew from

June and it's September now. What? You felt I couldn't be trusted?' Bubs sounded hurt.

'I was trying to get a hold on the whole thing myself.'

'So what you gonna do?' Bubs stood up to face him. 'You can't keep this shit up forever. Hell I'd hate to be in your shoes when you tell Claire.'

Ben turned away and paced the room uneasily. 'Kat says she can't live like this anymore. She wants me or she wants out.'

'And what about your son? She expects you to just forget about him?' Bubs pressed.

'He's her biggest dream, Bubs. She's a sickle sufferer and thought she would never have kids. She believed in some kind of prediction made years before by some fortune teller, about me and her meeting and having a child.'

'Claire is going to crucify your arse. About prediction and fortune teller! Another woman has your son? I told you this would grow beyond your control... Man, are you up shit street. When are you going to tell her?'

Ben had no intention of revealing Shadrach's existence to his wife; he considered it to be too cruel. Neither did he want to distress Kat any further. The Professor's words lay heavy in the pit of his gut like lead. He hadn't given any serious thoughts as to how many people would be hurt by this, and the Professor's disappointment in him gave his mind no peace.

'I'm not.'

'You have to. You can't continue living in cuckoo land, Ben. The reason Kat wants you to choose is because she wants to move on with her life. Man up, you owe it to her and Claire to tell her your decision. Now go because every time I see you lately, you confuse the fuck out of me.'

He drove home deep in thought. The tension was so stiff in his gut that he knew he had to sort his life out. It would mean seeing Kat again, telling her... telling her what? He did not know what he would say, not to Kat and not to Claire. His inner world was totally mired in confusion that was slowly, but surely submerging him.

He pulled into the driveway of his Chiswick home, parking his Mercedes alongside Claire's Saab. Her Mini Cooper was missing so that meant she was out. The oak door opened and Kenya stood bare feet waving in her Paddington Bear pyjamas. She was always the one to greet him as soon as she heard the car engine come up the drive.

'Daddy!' She jumped into his arms.

'Hi, pumpkin.' He carried her and his brief case into the house.

In the spacious living room, India sat on the L-shaped sofa, casually switching the television from station to station. 'Hi, Daddy,' she waved as he lowered Kenya onto the sofa beside her and dropped his brief case.

'Hello, beautiful, where's your mother?'

She shrugged her shoulders without taking her eyes of the television. 'She's probably at her Lupus meeting.'

'Hello, Ben.' Auntie Joan came into the room. 'Would you like your dinner now? You look shattered, everything okay?' Auntie Joan had always been receptive to his moods, since childhood.

He gave a pensive smile. 'Heavy day,' he told her. 'Any idea where Claire is?'

Aunty Joan suddenly looked worried. 'No, but I

think she's on the war path. She took a phone call and slammed out of the door as if she'd been given her death sentence.'

'Probably heard she missed out on a Gucci sale.'

They both laughed.

'You sure you don't want anything to eat?' Auntie persisted.

'Quite sure. I just need a shower... a brandy and coke would be great, just leave it in the study, I have some work to finish off.'

'You do look tired, Ben... sure there's nothing weighing heavy on your mind?'

'You know me so well.' He smiled, giving nothing away and headed upstairs for the shower.

The moon was so full and so bright that it looked as though it was sat just outside his study window. It looked fragile and paper-like and awesome. His thoughts were drawn to Kat again because he knew she would be mesmerised by such a sight and that something pertaining to the supernatural power of the universe would be called into debate. He laughed because it was her kind of crazy. He looked for the third time at his mobile phone sitting on the desk. He wanted to call her, to hear that Jamaican banter but knew he would only get a mechanical voice telling him to leave a message. He thought often too of his son, the chuckling, chubby baby who looked at him from familiar eyes—eyes that stared back at him whenever he looked in the mirror or at his youngest daughter.

'Daddy, why are you sad again?' It was Kenya, entering his study with a Pooh Bear teddy draped under one arm. Her eyes were sleep heavy and he knew she would fight the inevitable stealer of consciousness all the way. He held out his arms, needing to feel her small arms around his neck, her soft cheeks on his.

'You should be in bed,' he softly scolded, pulling her in close. She smelled of sweet soap and baby powder.

'Why are you sad, Daddy?'

He was astonished to know that his now six-year-old daughter had picked up on his unrest, but then Kenya was tuned into him.

'There you are, I should have known I'd find you with your daddy. It's bedtime,' Auntie Joan beckoned from the opened door.

'Night-night, pumpkin, sleep tight.' He kissed her before she obediently headed towards the door.

'Night-night, Daddy, don't let the bed bugs bite.'

It was way past midnight when Ben finally left the study and headed upstairs to bed. There was still no sign of Claire and it struck him as odd that she hadn't even called. He picked up his mobile phone and called her number. It rang until the voicemail kicked in. He left a simple message: 'Hey, dirty-stop-out, you forget you have a husband and two baby ducklings?'

Claire, Helen and her other friends, he knew, would be having fun no matter where they were. He was suddenly feeling tired and as soon as he climbed between the sheets, sleep accompanied him.

It was that feeling of not being alone, of being watched that made him start twisting and turning in the bed. So great was it that he began feeling tormented and it was this agony that finally jolted him upright out of his sleep. His eyes took a few seconds to adjust in the darkness, but when they did, he saw the outline of a figure standing in front of his bed. He turned to switch on the bedside lamp and Claire was there, her eyes dark and red rimmed, her mouth a pouty sulk.

'Claire!' He was startled and reached for her.

She backed away. 'Why would you do this to me, why?'

Her words stopped him in his tracks. 'Claire, what is it?' He looked towards the clock on the wall to see it was 03:15am.

'I've been thinking and thinking and working things out... how it all happened.' She was rambling but kept her sad, teary eyes on him. 'How stupid am I!' she spat angrily.

He became aware that she had been drinking because her body swayed with the movement of intoxication and the smell of alcohol had now penetrated his nose. She was no good at holding her liquor, but loved to drink anyway.

'Did you drive home in that state—'

'Shut up, shut up, just shut the fuck up!' she bellowed.

Ben became alarmed. 'What is it, Claire?'

'You should fucking know.' She suddenly switched to sarcasm: 'It's not nice not knowing, is it?' Her smile was frosty.

'I think we should get you some strong black coffee, then a few hours' sleep might just see you right.' He kicked the sheets off and made to get up. Claire could sometimes come home a little worse for drink. Alcohol made her merry and horny, she would normally want sex and more sex, not a fight and not at this hour of the morning.

Tears escaped and she impatiently brushed them away as though something disgusting had rolled down her cheeks. 'You... you hurt me, Ben. You've hurt me so badly. You've destroyed me.'

He felt at a total loss. 'Sweet girl.' He got up and moved towards her but she backed away. 'Claire, what is it?'

She glared at him silently.

'What's happened? Talk to me, come and sit.' He patted the bed beside him, trying to figure out what would make her behave like this, trying not to give in to the possibility that she might know. What else could make her behave this way? Yet she couldn't know, he told himself. She couldn't.

'What happened to you, baby, are you alright?'

She put both hands up, as if she was stopping an assault. 'Don't fucking talk to me.'

Yesterday morning when he had left for work she was in great spirits. They had made love and she even promised him more of the same later. He could not think what had upset her this much.

She withered to the floor, her coat forming a pool around her. 'You told me it was all in my head and I believed you. All I ever wanted was for our lives to be good, to give you children... give you the son you longed for... the son my ectopic took away any chance of... the son you now have with some fucking woman in Jamaica,' she screamed, her lips quivering, tears and the contents of her nose making a river into her mouth.

Ben froze. 'What?' His heart raced. She knew, how? Only Bubs and the Professor had that knowledge and he felt sure neither would have betrayed him in such a cruel way.

As if reading his thoughts she answered him, 'A woman called. She says she's the grandmother of your son... she called to say your son was sick in hospital... your son! I hope he dies.' She broke off weeping and sobbing, gripping her abdomen. 'I hope he fucking dies.'

It dawned on him then. He must have given Miss Ruthie the card with his home number on, not his mobile. But Shadrach was ill? His mind became splintered with chaos. He needed to speak to Kat, to Miss Ruthie, to someone who could tell him about his son's condition. He leapt out of the bed and headed downstairs to the study and all the time Claire was screaming behind him, words too riddled with pain to be coherent and his heart was breaking for her. The only number he now had was the Meadow's Post Office. He would ring it all night long if he had to; until someone answered and told him his son was okay.

Forty

Ben

He was okay, Shadrach was okay. Ben breathed a sigh of relief after finally getting through to the post office. A very curious, nosy, if he were honest, woman told him the baby was now home and that everyone in Miss Ruthie's household was well. She said her name was Miss Nellie and the name seemed to strike a familiar cord, though he could not remember why.

He eventually made his way back up to his bedroom, only to find the door locked. He didn't persist; he turned around and headed back to his study. It had all turned out wrong, so wrong and he was remorseful for what he had done to his wife and Kat. They had both suffered in this and he could only blame himself.

A troubled sleep claimed him again in the early hours of that Sunday morning, his arms serving as a pillow on his desk. He had no idea about what would happen next and for the first time in many years he felt aimless.

'Ben, Ben,' his head rose towards the soft soothing voice. He was reluctant to open his eyes because the sleep held on for so long, but the voice continued calling him, then a gentle shake finally made him sit up. It was

Auntie Joan, her face softened by concern.

'Is everything alright?' she enquired but her voice said she knew it wasn't. Her strong, plump hand guided his head to rest on her bosom where he had found so much comfort as a troubled child.

'You know, Ben, above all, be true to thy self. If God brought you to it He'll see you through it.'

Her kind and wise words always had an effect on him and this time was no different, he opened up his heart and told her the whole story, not stopping until it was all out, including the blame he solely took for the position the mothers of his children were in.

'It seems you have bitten off far more than you can ever chew,' she told him.

His arms went around her waist, and he held on, extracting comfort. 'I thought I could do this, I thought I could work it out so that no-one got hurt; now I've wrecked Kat's life and destroyed Claire's.'

Auntie Joan's fingers followed the trail of braids down his head.

'It is a very painful thing for all involved,' she told him, 'but the thing to do now is concentrate on the solution, not the problem.'

When Auntie Joan left to prepare breakfast for the children it was after 9am. He slowly pulled himself together knowing the first thing he must do was try to speak to Claire again. Before he could ease out of the chair, his mobile rang. He really didn't feel like talking to anyone but at the same time he welcomed the distraction.

'Ben, Ben are you alright?' The familiar voice, the musical banter caressed his ear.

'Kat!' He was overjoyed to hear her. He quickly pulled his thoughts together. 'How are you? How's Shaddy? Is he okay?'

'He's fine, a touch of pneumonia—but he's doing okay. You've certainly given Nellie Potato enough to keep her chewing for a while, calling at that unearthly time. She's acting as though she's saved Shaddy's life.' There was laughter in her voice. 'If anything bad had happened, I would have called so don't let anything worry you... are you okay?'

'Sure,' he lied, 'but Miss Ruthie called—'

'What possessed you to give her your number? Is all well at home? Did she cause any problems because I nearly died when she told me she'd left a message.'

'Everything's fine,' he lied again. 'Just as long as you and Shaddy are okay.'

'So how did you explain Miss Ruthie's message?' It sounded like a demand. 'Was it–it... who answered the phone? Who got Miss Ruthie's message?'

'Auntie Joan. Everything is fine, honest.' He had no idea why at this stage of chaos he was still deceiving, but this wasn't Kat's problem, it was his.

'I see you haven't called me.' She laughed nervously.

'I've been doing a lot of thinking.' He sounded awkward. 'I'm so sorry, Kat. I love you. I wish I could turn the clock back and change a few things.'

'Are you telling me goodbye?'

'No! I've made no decisions... I only know I love you, but—'

The phone went dead as her credit ran out. At least that's what he told himself, it was better than thinking she hung up.

Claire was in no mood to speak and the bedroom door remained firmly locked. He took his shower in the spare bathroom then tried his room door again. This time it was open but she was nowhere in sight. He dressed in blue tracksuit bottoms and a white polo shirt and headed downstairs.

'Daddy, can you help me with my project?' India met him as he entered the dining room.

'Okay, girls. Let's help India first, then what about if we go out for lunch this afternoon, we'll take Auntie Joan with us.'

The girls' squeals of delight were answer enough for him.

It took longer to finish India's project than expected because Kenya had to be kept occupied at the same time. When it was completed to her satisfaction, Auntie Joan took them to get dressed and they all headed out for lunch, at their favourite Caribbean restaurant in Portobello Road. He spoilt them, allowing them anything they wanted, to their utter surprise. But then he knew what lay ahead over the following months as he sought to mend the enormous crack he had created in their lives, a crack they were still unaware of. After lunch they went to the West End and walked around the toy shops, Ben giving in and allowing Kenya to choose yet another Pooh Bear, before also giving in to India's begging for Nike Huarache trainers. They arrived home after 8pm, the children tired but very happy. As he drove in the driveway, he saw that Claire's father's car was parked there. He was expecting it. They couldn't have a serious argument that her mother wouldn't want to get involved with.

In the living room, Claire sat forlorn, her arms folded and legs crossed, her eyes deliberately avoiding his. Sitting beside her was her mother, Jolene, huff and starchy, and opposite reading a heavy book was her father, Albert. He was a slim, trim man, his nutmeg skin tone creaseless, belying his age, and he would have a full head of hair, but he had always preferred short to the scalp cut, except for the periods during the 70s when he donned an afro, and he would tell that tale fondly.

Her mother was as usual, elegantly dressed in a lime green suede trouser suit and white silk shirt. Her dyed auburn hair and her red painted nails were the result of a beauty salon visit and the look on her face, the product of Claire's distress. Albert was the total opposite. His checked suit, although smart was worn and ancient; he had all his double-breasted suits made in the seventies and had seen no reason to update them. He often boasted that he had not gained an inch on his waistline.

'Grandpapa!' The girls greeted their grandfather first, rushing into his arms as he laughed and tickled them.

'We went to Portobello for lunch, then Daddy took us shopping down the West End,'

Kenya held up her Pooh Bear, 'I chose this and India got trainers.'

'That was very thoughtful of Daddy,' he said, squeezing her cheek.

'Hello, Grandmamma.' India kissed her grandmother's cheek formally, moving to one side so that Kenya could do the same.

'Glad you girls had a good time,' their grandmother

forced a smile.

'Come now, girls, let's get you washed; you look a mess.' Auntie Joan steered them out of the room before giving Ben a supportive smile.

The silence was illuminated by his mother-in-law's disapproval. Ben looked at Claire, who kept her head unnaturally straight, ignoring him. Albert went back to reading his heavy book, only Jolene viewed him with blatant distaste. It was she who finally broke the silence.

'Is this correct what we are hearing, Thornton? You've been having some affair with a–a Jamaican woman who now has your son?'

Ben viewed Claire as he answered with measured caution. 'With respect, Jolene, this is between Claire and me... I'm married to her.'

'There, there. Just like I said, now let's go and leave these kids to sort out their own problems, Jolene,' Albert quipped, giving Ben a sympathetic glance.

Ben would have given his father-in-law a grateful smile; only he knew it would be like offering a drowning man a glass of water. Jolene however was not having it. She stood to her elegant feet, tall and foreboding, her head bobbing like a spitting cobra.

'Bertie, I think we should support our daughter through this. She's devastated, her life ruined and all because her husband couldn't keep his trouser zipped up on so called business trips to Jamaica!'

Ben stood his ground. Their entire married life had been closely scrutinised by Jolene and it was about time he told her to butt out. 'As I said, Jolene, this is between Claire and me and I would thank you if for once in your life you could leave us to sort things out.'

Jolene took a step closer to him menacingly. 'Don't you dare speak to me like that you–you peasant! My daughter is too good for you.' Turning to Claire with a wagging finger she admonished her severely. 'I warned you about marrying someone with no family history, for all we know his father could have been a pimp, murderer or rapist and his mother a drug-taking prostitute, why else would they abandon him!'

That sent Ben reeling. It was way below the belt, even for Jolene. Claire looked horrified. Albert shut his book with a thud. He looked angrily at his wife before standing up.

'Ben is absolutely right—this is none of our business and you have no right saying those dreadful things. Claire,' her father turned to her; 'talk to your husband, not your mother. This is not her fight; it's yours, the fight for your marriage, your life. I don't condone what Ben has done, my darling,' a brief shadow of disapproval fleeted across his face, 'but that's life and that's relationships and the issue here is what you are both going to do next? Is this really past fixing? Give yourselves time, don't rush anything you'll probably regret later—'

'Bertie!' Jolene spoke to her husband angrily. 'I can't believe you're saying those things.' Then turning to her daughter she spoke softly, 'No second chances. Bring the children and come home; you don't have to put up with deceit in your marriage.'

'Jolene! Claire's is at home. Now let's go, leave them to it. There's nothing we can do here.'

At that point Albert picked up his book, his hat and his car keys. 'You coming, Jolene? Only I'm not waiting a moment longer.'

'But Bertie, we can't leave—'

'Then I'll see you when you get home... goodnight, Ben.' Albert nodded in Ben's direction. 'Claire, you think carefully now.' He held out the arm without the book and she ran to him. Tears pricked Ben's eyes at her heartbreak, the way she held onto her father like a frightened little girl. Albert placed a kiss on her forehead. 'You'll be stronger at the end of this, no matter what happens,' his voice was soft with kindness, 'and slow down on the drinking if you're to think straight. I know you love your husband and want your marriage to work, so find a way. See you soon.'

Jolene looked exasperated. 'We'll talk in the morning,' she told Claire, kissing her cheek before hurrying after her husband.

Claire poured herself another drink. She walked back over to the sofa and flopped down, taking a large sip.

'Now I understand it,' she said, looking at her half-empty glass. 'Those far away moments you're always having, then you wanting to convince me to do Jamaica instead of Italy. How the fuck would you have worked that out? That's my question.'

Ben couldn't look at her.

'You weren't even bothered if we didn't make love for weeks. All the time I thought you were considering my feelings about the ectopic.' She stood and made her way to pour another drink.

Ben frowned. 'I never lost my desire for you, not for a minute—'

'So, what's she like, this Jamaican girl?'

'Claire, I am so sorry, so sorry to hurt you like this.'

She laughed, loud and bitter. 'I don't believe you.

Tell me about her, I deserve to know that much.'

'There's nothing to tell, it won't solve anything.'

Claire shone with incredulity. 'What did you say?'

He reached for her hand but she slapped his attempt away.

'Don't touch me, Ben, don't fucking touch me. What are you saying?' She was totally disbelieving.

'Claire—' his voice trailed as her eyes, brimming with pain penetrated him.

'You have a son with another woman and there's nothing to tell?'

'Claire, please.' It was a whisper.

'Are you sure the child is yours?'

'Yes,' he said simply.

'How could you do that to me? You've split me open, my husband.'

He closed his eyes briefly, her words a hot rod through his head. 'Sweet girl, I didn't set out to—'

'After what happened to me you went out and got yourself a son? That's so cold.'

'It just wasn't like that.'

'You betrayed me.' She started to cry, then held on to the sob. 'Why? I mean, all that time. I even spoke to you about Taylor and Leon... thinking how lucky I was to have you, that our marriage was strong... and all the time you were betraying me, sleeping with another woman, giving her your child like I don't exist... oh God, what did I do?'

He bowed his head. 'I'm not proud of myself right now, and it's no use asking for forgiveness now either. But if–if you can just–just give me some time—'

'You need time to think whether you want us or not?

Are you fucking serious? Is that what you need time for?'

Ben looked up, his hands clasped together. 'No. I need to go to Jamaica, Claire, I need to go and see my son—'

'Fuck you! I don't believe you, I think you want to go and see her, and I can't take that Ben, you can't expect me to. No, no, no; if you go, then stay the fuck away. Don't come back home. You've got to leave me.'

Ben hated himself. He took a hesitant step towards her, gingerly. He was surprised she allowed him to take her hand. He turned it over and kissed the soft skin on her palm.

'I can't do that. I love you.'

Forty-one

Kat

'So, what will it be?'

Kat sat on her throne under the palm trees looking across the vast sea. The Pelicans were walking along the shore, their heads constantly dipping as their beaks sought washed-up treats deposited by the waves on to the sand. She turned to look at her baby son, his legs dangling over Columbus's shoulders, his little hands banging on Columbus's head as though he were playing a drum. Shadrach laughed when he looked at his mother and she made a funny face. The sun had already set and soon it would be time to head home. As they stood up, Columbus reached for her hand and gently repeated the question, 'Kat, *mon amour, veux-tu m'épouser?* Will you? Will you marry me?'

She sighed. 'Oh, Col, I'm not sure it's the right thing to do... you deserve real, real love.'

'I have all I need... you and Shaddy are more than enough.'

'Your problem is you've never been loved up the way a woman should love a man, or you wouldn't think that way.' She laughed to lighten the mood which had become far too heavy and serious. It was an alien place to be; having to seriously consider marriage to Columbus when she was still waiting on Ben's decision. She had to be sure it was really all over and that he was choosing to stay with his wife. And that was not what he said the last time she spoke with him. He'd said he loved her, he wanted her and she was frustrated with this answer because there was no conclusion.

Columbus lifted Shadrach off his shoulders and placed him on the sand.

'Look, I know you can't love me the way... the way you love Shaddy's father. I don't expect you to, but he's back with his wife and family now and there's no reason why you shouldn't find happiness too. I won't make any demands on you,' he said meaningfully. 'We are good friends and I just want us to give Shaddy a family life with a mum and dad... he deserves it, Kat.'

'You deserve more, Col, you can't settle for the little I can give you. You need to have your own baby with someone who loves you world without end. If we married, you would just end up hurt again.'

It was true. She knew she had hurt him. Her pregnancy had been devastating. When she told him, brimming with happiness that she was pregnant he had looked betrayed. For even though their relationship had been void of the desire that keeps lovers ignited, she knew he was satisfied being around her, soaked in her attention and flattered by her obvious adulation of his knowledge and his difference. No-one who knew the truth about their relationship understood. When the folks of the Meadows got hold of the news that Kat Lewis was expecting a baby, they all presumed it was for the white foreigner. After all they were inseparable for at least five months of the year over a ten-year period.

He reached out and touched her cheek. 'We should try, Kat. I love Shaddy like my own, I'll be the best step-daddy going and when the time comes to tell him about his real father, I will not object.'

'I don't want to spoil our friendship; you'd end up getting frustrated with me and even hate me... I couldn't stand it if you hated me, Col.'

His passion was total. '*Ma chérie*, I could never, ever hate you.'

'What about sex? You're young; you're going to need sex.'

The thought creased his forehead. 'Don't worry about that, I can promise you that I will make no demands. If I need to, I know where I can go for that.'

Kat's eyes widened with amazement, a smile spreading itself across her mouth. 'You are a dark horse, Columbus Jean-Paul McGregor... for the first time since I've known you I can truly say you've surprised me.'

He laughed. 'So... you going to give it a try?'

'Let me think about it.' She reached for Shadrach, opening his tiny hands to release the sand he had grasped. 'Miss Ruthie would want a big church wedding where she can invite the whole Christian Meadows.'

The smile on his face said it all. 'Are you saying yes?'

She contemplated the thought of it all. 'No, not yet.'

'I'll go with that.'

Kat saw that Miss Ruthie and Old Man were deep in conversation on the veranda in rocking chairs as Columbus pulled up in his jeep. The evening was warm and airless and Miss Ruthie could be seen fanning Old

Man with a folded newspaper. Around the light bulb on the veranda, dozens of little insects danced and in the distance the croaking of frogs sounded too close.

'I won't come in tonight, you look shattered.' Columbus smiled, placing a peck on her cheek.

'Good idea.'

He got out, opening the door for her, Shadrach sleeping soundly in her arms.

'See you tomorrow,' he kissed her forehead. '*Merci*... thanks, Kat, for even considering this.'

After Shadrach had settled down for the night, Kat joined Miss Ruthie and Old Man on the veranda with glasses of ice cold lemonade.

'It will rain tomorrow,' Old Man said, 'it way too hot, the heat must break... it's winter and still so hot, this is not like it use to be.'

'It must be the environment thing you always talking about,' Ruthie pointed out.

Kat sat opposite them and handed the lemonade.

'Global warming. The whole earth is warming up and doing unusual things,' she stated.

Miss Ruthie filled her mouth with rice from the small brown bag on her lap.

'God Almighty soon take back him earth, mankind too ungrateful,' she prophesised between chews. 'What riding you mind?'

Kat laughed at her mother's intuition. 'Columbus asked me to marry him.'

'He's done that before,' she huffed.

'This time I said I'd think about it.'

'You mad or something?'

Kat viewed her in surprise. 'I thought you'd be happy, Miss Ruthie. You're always telling me to marry him.'

Miss Ruthie sighed, her body shrinking as she looked to Old Man. 'I can sometimes be wrong,' she confessed.

Kat was truly puzzled. 'Are you saying you don't want me to marry Col?'

Old Man squeezed her hand. 'If you love him, do. But don't marry him as an alternative. It not good. True love mus' be present for a marriage to work.'

'Col loves me... a whole heap—'

'You love him? Like, real love?' Old Man's question was soft, but thumped her hard.

Her silence said it all.

'Then don't do it. Marry the man you love,' he smiled kindly.

Tears filled her eyes unexpectedly. She was annoyed with herself. If she were to tell that Ben was married, then she would have another mêlée on her hand, Miss Ruthie would be caught up in recrimination and acute disappointment, not to mention the reels of prayers she would parade. Kat just did not have the energy or the inclination for such a battle.

'I don't love Col like Ben, Old Man, but he'll make a good father, he'll take care of us.'

'If you mean him any good, then you need to love him like a man... a man can walk more miles when he know he have a woman who love him, love him like a man, not a friend or a brother, like a man.' His smile settled on Miss Ruthie.

Kat stood to her feet snappishly. She needed a distraction from Ben, her longing for him, the conflict that seized her. Columbus helped her overcome confusion, and maybe he would eventually help her conquer the love that burned too deep and had left a huge crater in her life. She didn't know what to do.

'I need help, Miss Ruthie,' she said earnestly. 'I need help.'

Forty-two

Ben

London

Ben drove in silence through the traffic on Chiswick High Road, as he headed towards Fulham to drop the children off at their private Seven Day Adventist Church School. He hadn't slept. He couldn't shake Claire's devastation from his mind. It had wounded him to the core. In hindsight he should have expected it and prepared for it.

'Hey, Daddy, keep your eyes on the road.' India prodded him.

'Sorry, girl.'

He dropped the children off knowing he must explain to them about their brother before the end of the week.

The working day progressed slowly as he battled for concentration. This was his burden to bear, consequences caused by his actions. How he had dreaded the day when he would have to face reality and make choices that would change his world. Decisions he delayed in the hope that things would work themselves out, that somehow a miracle would happen and Claire would accept his love for Kat and they would all live happily. Now he wondered where his mind had got this notion from. Or even more absurd, how he managed to convince his usually logical brain to entertain such thoughts and believe them. Kat made him feel all things were possible, as did Claire. He was torn. No, he didn't want to hurt Claire any more than he already had, but he struggled to give up the thought of Katherine Lewis. There would be a place for her within his very being for eternity and he didn't know how to shake that, to dislodge and dissolve it into obliteration. His calm in all of this came from his children, including Shadrach. They anchored his thoughts whenever hopelessness overwhelmed him.

'Daddy! Where's Auntie Joan?' Kenya asked excitingly at seeing her father sat in his car outside the iron school gates.

'I told her I'd pick you girls up; spend some father-daughter time together, go eat some place, what d'you think?'

Kenya squealed in delight and jumped in the back. India was cool about the idea.

'Oh, Daddy, I wanted to go round Tilly's tonight so we can watch *Sex and the City*. Why do we need to eat out? Isn't Auntie Joan cooking?'

'You watch what! Are you even old enough?'

'I watch it with Mummy all the time,' she announced with flippant importance.

Now wasn't the time to challenge Claire on this. He knew she would probably win, she had a mouth on her, one of the things he was attracted by. 'I thought we might eat at Saba's, the little Ethiopian restaurant in Richmond.'

'Okay.' India perked up, as her father knew she would.

Saba was her favourite restaurant where he had allowed her sips of honey wine to celebrate her tenth birthday. She had been badgering for a repeat ever since.

He watched his daughters as they ate and chatted about their school day. A stubborn knot had formed in his throat and no amount of swallowing was budging it. During the dessert, he broached the subject with caution, watching their little faces for any sign of disapproval or confusion.

'I have something to tell you both.'

Kenya remained uninterested but India looked concerned. 'What is it, Daddy?' India asked, her eyes fearful. 'Are you and Mummy getting a divorce, like Auntie Taylor and Uncle Leon?'

'Why would you think that?' Ben quizzed, a little uneasy about India being so informed about Taylor and Leon, but understanding fully that Claire was the type of mother who would not lie to her children and would answer all their questions.

'Coz you and Mummy didn't sleep together again last night,' Kenya announced, spooning a heap of chocolate cake into her mouth. 'India says so.'

India speared her sister with a look of displeasure. Ben put his fork down and viewed his daughters. It hadn't occurred to him that they would have noticed such things. He had made sure they were still in their beds before leaving the spare room in the morning.

'Mummy's not happy right now,' Ben spoke evenly. 'Something happened which is going to take some time getting used to for all of us.'

They were still more absorbed in their dessert than conversation.

'It's hard for you to understand this, but you have a baby brother, my son with another woman—'

'Daddy! You had an affair!' India's eyes opened in horror.

Ben turned his back as heads from surrounding tables turned to view him, some with outright disapproval, others with surprise, amusement and perhaps disbelief.

'How could you? Does Mummy know?' India's babble, now lowered to a whisper as she realised people were staring at them, was clothed in displeasure.

'Yes,' he confessed ruefully.

'That's why Mummy's been so mad at you?'

Ben felt like the child answering to his parent. 'Yes. Now if you'll let me finish I have something important to tell you both. I have to go to Jamaica, just for a while, one week. I have to see Shaddy, your baby brother and sort things out.'

'You're leaving us? Me and Kenya?' India's eyes suddenly filled with fear.

'No, no, darling, I would never do that. You'll always be my girls.'

'So why do you need to see that baby? Can't you just send him some money and then leave him alone?'

Ben's cheeks ballooned with a sigh as he attempted to explain. 'I think it wouldn't be right to just forget about my child, your brother. I think he would grow up feeling rejected, like no-one loved him. What I've done has hurt people; I have to put things right. I hurt Mummy—'

'Did you tell her sorry?' Kenya asked.

He smiled at his youngest and wondered why we couldn't bring that simplicity of reasoning and problem solving into the adult world with us. 'Yes.'

They arrived home a little after 9pm.

The front door opened and Claire stood relieved.

Ben gave a weary smile. 'Hi, sorry we're so late.'

'Where have you been with my children? And why didn't you tell me you were taking them out?'

He realised she had been worried. 'You were sleeping. I told Auntie Joan to tell you.'

'Well she wasn't in when I woke up and I couldn't find the children and you didn't answer your phone... I thought, I thought you'd taken them, that you'd gone,' she started crying and the children ran to her, hugging her and apologising.

'We didn't mean to scare you, Mummy,' India was tearful too. 'Don't worry, we wouldn't leave you.'

'No, we wouldn't, sorry to put you through that, Claire. Come, girls, go get ready for bed, I'll be up to check on you, let Mummy and me have a talk.'

It was after midnight when Ben tried the bedroom door. He was surprised that it was not locked. Claire was sat up in bed staring blankly at the television screen. Her hair was in a bun, her eyes were swollen with the aftermath of uncontrollable tears and she looked clothed in total despair.

'Claire—'

'I don't want you sleeping in here... just leave me alone.'

He walked and stood in front of the plasma screen which occupied half of the wall.

'Sorry.'

She glared at him.

'Sorry, okay? Sorry. I don't know how many times

I can say it, but I'm sorry.' He walked towards her, his hand went out to stroke her face but she slapped him away.

'Don't. I can't bear you near me, Ben, just leave, fucking leave.'

'I understand how you feel. I've betrayed you, hurt you and I'm sorry. I know it sounds ridiculous, but there was no intentions to hurt you. I value our marriage and I can see by that look you think I'm talking shit, but I–I can't explain this in any way that you'll ever be able to understand.'

'Oh, I see. It's a man thing. A woman wouldn't be able to understand this higher intellect. A fucking male privilege crap thing of having your cake and eating it! Fuck off!'

With his hands deep in his pockets, he looked at her forlornly, overwhelmed by the misery she was in and he was causing.

'If you value our marriage so much, why did you fuck another woman? Why did you love her? Give her your son!' Claire cried.

'I don't know.' He shrugged his shoulders in hopeless resignation.

'Didn't I please you?'

'It's not about that, sweet girl, of course you please me.'

'Is she prettier than me? Better in bed? What did I lack? What wasn't I good at? What's wrong with me?'

'Don't do this... it's self-torture.' Sadness tainted his voice. 'There's nothing wrong with you—'

'So, it's my fault for torturing myself?'

'Okay, it happened and I'm sorry I hurt you—I'm

selfish and didn't think beyond my own needs. I confused myself, I disgust myself, I get angry, what can I tell you, Claire? Nothing I tell you can justify what I–I did... but I won't deny that I love you. I love you.'

'How will I ever trust you again?'

Ben sighed. 'Claire, we have the girls to think about, let's not rush, okay? Let's both have some reflection time.'

'You made love to another woman and gave her your son... and you continue to love her... to want her. Look in my eyes and tell me you don't. Tell me I'm all you need and want and that you'll never see her or that child again... tell me that and we can talk, reflect.'

Ben sighed and looked away. If he could, it might solve her pain and return some normality back to his life. But there were forces at work here that he had no understanding of. He only discovered that they existed through Kat.

'I won't lie to you again, Claire. I can promise you that.' He was unable to meet her eyes. There could be no more lies or deception, neither his conscience nor his heart would tolerate it.

'I never saw this coming, you know.' She sounded wounded.

'Let's talk about this.' He still wanted to fix what was broken. Life had changed, who he was had changed but he was still trying to hold on.

'It hurts me even to look at you,' she sobbed.

'I know.' Ben walked over to the window and stared out onto the frost-covered front lawn. He watched a squirrel, a nut of some kind clenched between its tiny hands as it nibbled away. How uncomplicated the life of a squirrel was. But then a squirrel knew nothing of the human emotion to love two women. How uncomplicated, he mused.

'Ben, if our marriage is to work then you have to promise never to see her or that child.'

When he turned back to face her, he saw her hold her breath at the look on his face.

'I can't. I have to see my son again; sorry, but surely you can see that. He's mine.' He clenched his fist to his heart. 'I've given him so little and I can't just abandon him, you must know that much about me. I'm not the kind of man who can turn my back on my own child, carrying on as though he doesn't exist... you know that if nothing else.'

'You love her more.' Claire stood transfixed before him, her eyes bright and accusing.

His silence stretched as he seriously considered this. Finally he said, 'More? No, no.' He shook his head vigorously. 'That's not true, that's just not true.'

Forty-three

Kat

Jamaica

Kat had just showered when her mobile rang. What she was not anticipating as she answered it was the unfamiliar, English female voice that she heard.

'Kat? Is–is this Kat?'

'Who wants to know?' Kat teased, laughing into the phone, believing her friend Paula was playing a trick on her.

The woman sighed heavily, impatient. 'Mrs Benjamin. Claire-Louise Benjamin.'

Kat's breath caught in her throat as her laughter melted. Her heart raced and a sick feeling twisted her stomach. Words failed her.

'Your silence tells me something,' Claire said coldly. 'I think we need to talk, don't you?'

How did she know? Had Ben's Auntie Joan told her about Miss Ruthie's phone call? Ben's wife on the phone wanting to talk. What could she say? What was Claire-Louise expecting? By her tone Kat could sense tension, concealed anger.

'Can you meet me in the bar area of Hotel Panama?'

Claire pushed.

Hotel Panama. Kat was stunned into even more silence. Was Claire-Louise in Jamaica, in the Meadows?

'Yes,' Claire answered Kat's thoughts. 'I'm here in Jamaica and I won't be going anywhere until I see you. Shall we say 6pm, that gives you two hours.'

Finally Kat found her voice. 'If you think it a good idea—'

'Yes, I do,' Claire snapped. 'Six. And please, don't mention this call or our meeting to my husband.' Then she swiftly hung up.

Kat sat on her bed looking from her mobile phone to the clock on her wall. Her mouth felt dry and her heart was still hammering, protesting at being given such a shock. Shadrach crawled into the room. His beaming smile, baby babbling and sparkling eyes reminded her of what she had, and what she would not have had without Ben. She picked up her son and hugged him close. 'I won't let anyone make me feel bad about you, baby boy.' She kissed his cheek and placed him down, laughing as he crawled back towards Miss Ruthie's singing.

Her phone rang and she sighed. It was Rosie.

'What a gwaan, girl?'

'Rosie, you will not believe who just phoned me.'

'Tell me,' Rosie said.

'Ben's wife... Claire-Louise,' she whispered, fully aware that Miss Ruthie was only yards away. 'She's here in the Meadows and wants to meet with me in two hours.'

'You want me come with you?' Rosie offered with relish.

Kat thought seriously about the offer for a moment

341

before rejecting it.

'Not a good idea. She might feel threatened and it will look too school girlish.'

'So,' Rosie said, 'you think you can handle it?'

'I have no choice.'

'Well just you remember that it's the lady's husband—go easy. Swallow all the shit she throw 'cos you and Candy Eyes are in the wrong. Just because you love each other don't make it right. You guys betrayed her and she knows it, so just be ready for anything. But if she throws a first punch, then you punch back, depending how big she is. If she's much bigger than you, use your feet to kick—it's stronger than our fists. Man I would love to be a fly on that wall.'

'Thanks,' Kat said gloomily before hanging up, 'you've been a great help.'

Kat turned out her limited wardrobe, tried on different dresses, jeans, T-shirts and felt close to despair at not finding anything suitable. What does one wear for a meeting with your lover's wife? Eventually she settled for her white linen dress which buttoned down the front and which Ben always said she looked good in. It had a stylish cut which enhanced her shape. Columbus had bought her a pair of Parisian lime green sandals with heels and matching bag, which went really well with a hair band Old Man had given her one birthday. She combed her hair and used the band to hold it out of her face. Then she slipped her feet into the heels and looked at herself in the mirror. Her hair needed a hairdresser. She was on the route of panic when Miss Ruthie came into the room, a sleeping Shadrach in her arms. 'You looking very pretty, I never know you going out,' she said, placing the baby in his cot.

'Rosie and I are just going to have dinner on the beach. I just feel to look different.' She stared at her reflection. 'What about my hair? You really think I look pretty, Miss Ruthie?'

'Very. I was wondering if you have a new beau, and nothing wrong with you hair.'

The sky had been washed orange by the outgoing sunset, nature's way of tempting an artist's creativity, she thought. She sat for a long time outside one of the shops on the beach rehearsing what she would say to Ben's wife, but failing miserably to find anything that didn't sound cliché. Finally she worked up some courage and caught the taxi to the town centre. It stopped outside the plush hotel Panama and one of the attendants immediately opened the car door for her to step out. She thanked him and walked nervously into the reception and then through to the bar and restaurant area.

She needed no introduction. Ben's wife stood out among the guests. She wore a sleeveless lilac dress which fitted her tall slender frame like a glove and accessorised it with matching pearl earrings, necklace and a bracelet. Her hair was cut with a fringe and fell past her shoulders. Kat wrestled with the feeling of inadequacy and would have turned and hurried out, but at that moment their eyes locked and she saw the flash of recognition that filled Claire's. Kat sat down, her clasped hands on her lap. No-one spoke for a long moment which stretched unbearably and it was the waiter who came to take orders that finally broke their stares. After the orders and the drinks were placed in front of them, Claire spoke.

'I saw you and instinctively knew it was you.'

Kat sipped her white wine before responding, 'Yes. I instinctively knew you too.'

'You're pretty... not what I imagined.'

'Thank you.'

'It's not a compliment,' Claire said, her voice flat and expressionless. 'I'm not here to be nice; I'm just stating a fact.'

'And you're very beautiful,' Kat spoke with measured tones.

Claire laughed. 'Not beautiful enough... not enough to stop my husband from playing out.'

Kat didn't respond. She knew she was there for at least two reasons, one of which was to satisfy Claire-Louise's curiosity, the other to take her insults. She was willing to do what Rosie had said and swallow the shit thrown at her. She accepted her part in this woman's devastation, but wasn't she devastated too?

'I suppose you want to know why I've asked to meet with you.' Claire sounded uptight. 'To be honest, I haven't a clue.' She took a big gulp of her drink and emptied the glass. 'Waiter.' She waved a perfectly manicured hand, painted with lilac nail varnish. 'Bring me the whole bottle of wine please,' she ordered. 'More wine?' she offered Kat stiffly.

'No, I'm not much of a drinker,' Kat admitted.

Claire finished another glass and refilled. 'Bit like my husband. Ben doesn't drink too much, he always tells me to slow down when we're out. It's a bit of a joke among my girlfriends how he counts my drinks. "Claire, sweet girl, go easy on the booze," he says. But what can I say, I like a drink and I don't apologise.'

So he calls her 'sweet girl' too. Kat felt a pang of jealousy. She looked around and saw that there were a few people left at the other tables. Mid-week at Hotel Panama was usually quiet, but unfortunately for her Nellie Potato's granddaughter, Su-Anna was one of the guests, sitting with her head resting on the shoulders of her very married boss.

'So, Kat.' Claire's voice was slightly raised as she continued to drink, at a slower rate now. 'I guess I wanted to see what you looked like, what my husband is willing to risk all for, and finally what your game is.'

'My game?' Kat queried.

Claire laughed. 'Yes. What are you up to, sleeping with a married man?'

Kat hung her head briefly. 'I didn't know that when we first met.'

Claire narrowed her eyes. 'What's your profession, if you don't mind me asking?'

Kat took a small sip from her glass. 'I'm an artist.'

Claire's eyes took on interest. 'You did that sketch of him, didn't you? The one he has in his office! Of course! Oh fuck! What's your initials; KL?'

Kat didn't have to respond.

'You've gone deep with my husband.' Claire took another sip. 'You captured him, my husband like I've never seen him... like he's a different man with you.'

Kat remained silent in her deepening anguish, seeing Ben's love—this beautiful woman—cut her in two.

'And your accent, it's not totally Jamaican, is it? Are you mixed with something? Your hair, it's—'

'Jamaican born and bred.' Kat was becoming impatient. 'And so is my mother and my father and all the family I know.' She wanted Claire to get on with whatever it was she was here to say so that she could go home and lick her wounds. 'Sorry to be rude, but can you get to the point? Why did you invite me here? What is it you want to really say?'

'Where's your child? I understand my husband is the father?' Claire's lips trembled and Kat knew she didn't want to be vindictive to this woman. She didn't want to cause her anymore pain than she already had.

'My son is at home with my mother,' she hesitated, 'and yes, Ben is his father.'

She saw Claire wince, refill her glass and look despairingly at it.

Kat continued, 'I don't know what you want me to say.' She looked directly into Claire's eyes. 'I know you don't want my apologies, and I won't patronise you with them. You've come a long way to confront me which tells me how much you love Ben. You're here to fight for him, to warn me off.' She pushed her glass away. 'I'll answer all your questions, if you listen to my side of things.'

Claire was visibly shaken. She fidgeted with her wedding band and instantly looked like a bewildered child. 'Do you love him?' Her voice was small and quivered with the weight of her tears.

Kat turned her head away, her own lips trembling with threatening tears.

'You promised to answer all my questions,' Claire pointed out.

'Yes,' Kat whispered. She saw the pain cut across Claire's face and wished she could have done things differently. 'Yes, I love him but I've also accepted our fate whatever it turns out to be.'

'Fate? You talk to my husband about... fate? Did you ask my husband to leave me and his children?'

'No!' Kat exclaimed.

Claire looked puzzled. 'But you say you love him. If you love him, why wouldn't you want him with you and your child? Was it a sexual thing for you? To have his child so you can claim an income, artists are badly paid, is that it?'

Kat shook her head hopelessly knowing anything she said would never be understood by Claire.

'For God's sake, you knew he was married! Didn't you wonder about me? About his children, before you opened your legs?'

Kat looked fiercely at Claire, took a deep breath and exhaled silently.

'I won't go to that level, Claire-Louise, I won't go that low. In an ideal world, yes,' Kat admitted, 'I should have kept my legs shut, as you put it—but we both know it's not an ideal world. I didn't force Ben into bed, I didn't put a gun or knife to his head and say "fuck me"—we wanted each other, he wanted me.'

'So that made it okay? Even though he was married with kids, you wanted each other so that's fucking that.' Claire supported her forehead with a hand, and when she looked up her mascara blackened eyes deepened her despair.

'... Why did you have to give him a child?' she asked in a broken hushed voice. 'Why not just fuck him and walk away? Why did you have to give him a son? I'm his wife, not you.' Claire went into her handbag and took out a small powder blue package which she pushed towards

Kat. 'This rightfully belongs to–to you, so whatever comes out here today, I don't hate your son or wish him any ill. There's no reason why you should believe me other than I'm asking, take it… please.'

For that second, Kat felt something surreal pass between them, and for no reason other than she felt she should, the sky blue package was in her hand and straight in her bag. She shivered and realised that the air conditioner had caused goose bumps to rise on her skin. She hated this artificial air and longed to go outside to feel the natural warmth of the evening sea breeze. She hated to see first-hand what their love, hers and Ben's had done to his wife. There was guilt, but there was also genuine love which cleared her conscience and she failed to summon regret. She loved Ben and she knew too that he loved her, so if there was any fault, any blame to be had it should be placed at the feet of fate. For it was fate with that tragic sense of humour, that twister, that stealer, that giver of life and dreams that had caused this. She looked at Claire and remembered Mother Cynthy's reading: An angry stranger.

'This is not personal; I have nothing against you—'

'It's what you have with my husband, that's the issue here, isn't it?'

Kat stood up. 'In another life, out of this situation I think I could have liked you and maybe you would have liked me too. I really don't think anything is going to be resolved by me being here and for what it's worth, I'm truly sorry to have caused so much distress.'

'But you did. That's the problem. You've changed my life forever and I don't even know you. Why didn't you leave when you knew he was married? Why?'

Kat stared steadily at her lover's wife. Rosie's words came back to her: *Loving each other don't make it right!*

'His love, it–it caught me. The way he is, warm, loving, thoughtful, funny, feels so good to be around. He cares about my heart—I don't need to tell you about your husband.'

Kat could see Claire was fighting for control. Her perfectly painted lips had lost their gloss and the glass dangling between her fingers bore a smudged print.

Claire stared back, her eyes coloured with pain. 'But you do, because I don't know the side you know. I don't know the Ben in that drawing... it caught so much, a picture paints a thousand words and that one painted more than a fucking thousand words.'

Kat lingered awkwardly; looking over her shoulder at the few customers at their tables who were obviously intrigued by Claire's slightly raised voice. Especially Su-Anna.

'I've gone against everything I believe in by loving Ben, there's no more to say.'

Kat wanted to leave the pained eyes that cornered her. Seeing her lover's wife had made everything far too real.

Claire stood up to face her, steadying herself against the table. The consumption of the alcohol had taken full effect. 'You need to say more—you broke my marriage,' Claire said tearfully.

'I wasn't the one lying to you—I didn't even know you, my loyalty was to Ben and–and when I met him he said he wasn't married. He's changed my life completely now, made me a mother and I can't lie and tell you I'm sorry about that,' Kat spoke calm, almost gentle.

'It wasn't my intention to hurt you. Had I known Ben was married right off, I would not have entertained the thought, whether you believe me or not. But once–once we got close, it wasn't so easy to leave him, to walk away and never see him again... I love him and I'm just sorry that–that it all turned out like this... but my son is everything and given the chance to do it all again... I would still want my son.'

'Well I'm here to tell you more... a lot more. I loved my husband long before you even knew he existed. Everything you've done with him, I've done it and a lot more. It kills me that he loves you, but I know he loves me, I know that!'

'Yes,' Kat nodded in agreement.

'But he's weak for you and so he needs my strength. You need to leave him because the truth is, he won't leave you because he's–' she broke off to laugh, 'he's loyal. He won't want to reject or abandon you, or me. He'll go on having you and me and you and me, pulling himself to pieces so not to disappoint, but destroying us all in the process–and I don't want that for my kids and I can't live like that, can you?'

Kat didn't answer; the truth was swirling too fast to shake for any authenticity–and its impact she did not want to face in front of her lover's wife.

'I love my husband and I'll fight you all the way. You will lose, son or not. I'm the only Mrs Benjamin.' She held up her ringed finger. 'I am the real Mrs Thornton Benjamin... so who the fuck are you?'

Kat took a step back, the film footage of her and Ben's relationship reeling through her mind. She wasn't going to let Claire leave believing that she, Kat, was nothing but a fling.

'Who am I? Someone important enough for you to travel four thousand miles to warn off. Your ring and your title didn't keep him from me, and that's why you're here... so I know my power, and now you know my power. Goodbye, Mrs Benjamin.'

Forty-four
Kat

Before she closed her eyes to sleep that night, Kat tried to contact Ben to tell him about her encounter with Claire-Louise. She had met his love, his wife, beautiful, stunning, sexy and broken. And to top it, folded neatly in the powder blue package was a miniature football kit, red, with 'Manchester United' boldly standing out. It would be at least a year before Shaddy could wear it, if she let him. It puzzled her that her lover's wife gave a gift to his son from another woman.

Unable to sleep she called Rosie and whispered everything that had taken place, and told her how it ended.

'She gave you what? Man U football kit for Shaddy... and still cuss you out... that strange... you better get it blessed before you put Shaddy in it. You know about them mad English people.'

'I really don't think she's like that... she's beautiful, Rosie. Her skin, her hair and I'm sure her smile is pretty, I just never saw it. She laughed, but it wasn't real laughter. Looking at her I kept wondering what Ben sees in me... she seems to have it all.'

'Yeah, it makes you wonder if a man can ever be satisfied. Was that a threat you left her with?' Rosie asked.

'No. I just wanted her to know that I'm important to Ben, he loves me too.'

'I think she knows that, you didn't have to rub it in.'

'I didn't, Rosie, I played it calm like you said. It was just at the end I felt she wanted to belittle me so I kicked back a little.'

'It's her husband, Kat. It's the woman's husband.'

Kat began crying into the phone. 'I know, Rosie, but I love him,' she sobbed passionately. 'And so does his wife. Oh Rosie, you should've seen her, I hated myself, and I felt so, so bad. I can't forget the look in her eyes when she asked if Ben was Shaddy's father, it broke her. And I don't understand that gift to Shaddy, but I'm thinking it has some significance. Ben should know. I'll ask him.'

'Your head is full,' Rosie told her, 'go get some shut eye and we talk in the morning.'

Kat hung up, swiftly drifting into a restless sleep.

The first customers of the day were Nellie Potato and Su-Anna, no surprise to Kat.

The relationship between herself and Nellie had been strained, cold even, since that day she had given the old woman a piece of her mind. No doubt Nellie had been waiting for the perfect opportunity to wreak revenge, and thanks to Claire-Louise, she got her perfect chance.

Miss Ruthie had hardly finished setting up the provisions and Kat had just put food out for Samson when the familiar squeak of the gate made them both look up. Kat exhaled hard. If she could have requested any gift from God it would have been the gift of hindsight. For she now knew that with hindsight she would have revealed everything to Miss Ruthie from the beginning.

Kat watched the two women, one old, the other young walking with an unnatural air of confidence, her secret now known by them. She thought of going inside, of busying herself. Her only fear was the grief, disappointment and embarrassment she knew her mother would feel and she wished with all her heart that she could save Miss Ruthie from what was about to be revealed to her.

'Morning, Miss Rootie,' Nellie Potato spoke first. 'Trusting that the good Lord will bless you on this fine, fine day.'

Miss Ruthie mumbled a response.

'Good morning, Miss Rootie,' Su-Anna spoke but her eyes were on Kat.

Miss Ruthie noticed. 'Su-Anna!' she exclaimed. 'What wind blew you this way? I not seen you here for months.'

Nellie Potato didn't wait for her grand-daughter's response. 'We come to speak with you, Miss Rootie... to tell you something important... something Su-Anna see with her own eyes which you should know long time but I think people bin lying to you.' Her eyes rolled lingeringly over Kat, her smirk revealing how much she was enjoying her newfound power.

Miss Ruthie looked at Kat, puzzled. Kat stood frozen to the spot, thoughts thrown around in her head like clothes in a tumble dryer.

'Nellie Potato,' Ruthie took a deep breath, 'you know I don't want no su-su talk at my head this time of morning. Too much to do and I have Old Man to prepare breakfast for.'

The knowing smile that played around Nellie's mouth was quite sinister and Kat could see Miss Ruthie was concerned. There was no doubt that Nellie Potato still had beef to grind with Kat. The whole of the Meadows knew that Kat's verbal outburst at Nellie had left her bitter. Everyone who entered the post office was given her version and interpretation of Miss Ruthie's disrespectful and bad breed child's attack on her.

Nellie Potato's eyes, mouth, the twist of her body, the words that came with the piercing sharpness of a knife would accompany Miss Ruthie to the end of her days. 'Beg your pardon, Miss Rootie,' Nellie said. 'This is not su-su,' she turned towards Kat, 'is it, Kat?'

Kat was not saying anything.

'Your mother don't know, does she?' Nellie's teasing was transparent. 'You who cuss me out, disrespect me in front of people! You! You are a demon from hell!'

And still Kat said nothing as Miss Ruthie became increasingly confused. Nellie continued, 'Su-Anna was in Hotel Panama yesterday, and she see with her own eyes and overhear with her own ears, Kat.'

Kat, for the first time in her life, could not look at her mother. She didn't want to see the shame she knew would appear, the devastation. And worst of all, Nellie Potato, her mother's nemesis had this power over her. She wished Old Man was his old self. He would have heard the commotion, but his mobility would not allow him to come out unaided.

Miss Ruthie spoke to Kat, 'You want to tell me or you want Nellie Potato tell me?' Her voice contained a calm that was denied her mind. Kat finally looked up at her mother, her eyes, dark pools of misery and remorse.

'Kat!' Miss Ruthie showed the alarm that struck her.

Nellie Potato laughed. 'Your mouth not so big now! Huh! You disrespect your elders and think God Almighty wouldn't punish you?'

'Kat!' Miss Ruthie demanded.

'Miss Ruthie, let's go inside. I'll explain.'

'Explain what?' Nellie Potato moved very quickly for someone who had so many ailments, Miss Ruthie thought. Nellie stood in front of her, looking from her to Kat. 'That you fornicated with a woman's husband, had your child in sin and that the woman come all the way from foreign to find you and cuss you out! Right there in Hotel Panama! Su-Anna see it all! She make a baby with a married man, some foreign woman's husband. She bring shame and scandal on your house, Miss Rootie, shame and scandal... open your door to Satan—'

'Stop! Stop right now!' Miss Ruthie's voice was harsh and loud, louder than anyone had ever heard. The mist was weighty and suffocating as it descended and wrapped itself around her. 'Nellie Potato, your words are like a knife twisting in my womb. I thank you to keep your opinions to yourself. I will conduct my own affairs.'

'But Miss Rootie—' Nellie's voice momentarily trailed at the sharp look Miss Ruthie gave her. 'It must hurt, I know Miss Rootie, but the truth is an offence, but not a sin. I can only say the devil possess these women who fornicate with a next woman's husband—'

'You could be right, Nellie Potato,' Old Man interjected from the door. He was still in his pyjamas and

356

leaning heavily on his walking stick. 'Let Miss Rootie take care of her possessed child and you go take care of your possessed grandchild. She fornicating with her boss, Miss Edwina's husband... been fornicating with him for years,' Old Man focused on Su-Anna, who was now inching her way back to the gate, guilt blatant on her face. 'Have you told your grandmother, Su-Anna? You tell her how many 'bortions you have? And while you at it, Nellie Potato, you go see what your husband, Farmer Tom up to with Sister Pam.'

Kat could have kissed Old Man there and then. She didn't know that he knew about Su-Anna. The thought had crossed her mind to get angry and focus on Su-Anna's affair, but in a way she was glad that Miss Ruthie now knew about Ben.

If looks could kill then Su-Anna would be deader than the dead as thunder struck Nellie Potato's face. She looked murderously at Kat. 'This don't excuse your evil ways. You destroyed a family sanctified by God—'

'And so has Su-Anna. Now you go take care of your devil.' Old Man looked towards Kat. 'And Miss Rootie will take care of hers.'

As Miss Ruthie helped Old Man to wash and dress, and after he ate his breakfast and went to sit on the veranda, Kat prepared Shadrach's bath, knowing she would eventually have to face her mother. How she was glad that Old Man had been there, his vibrant optimism, his outrageous wisdom, Miss Ruthie needed them.

Kat settled Shadrach in his chair with his bottle. The room felt heavy with Miss Ruthie's disapproval. A well of emotions seeped to Kat's throat and she found it impossible to get the words out without the tears first erupting. Miss Ruthie continued in her silence, ignoring the tears that streamed down her daughter's face.

'I'm... so sorry... I didn't want Nellie Potato telling you.'

Miss Ruthie's voice was quiet and shaky. 'Why?' she pleaded. 'Why you fornicate with a married man? Are you possessed?'

Kat knew her mother was serious and expected an answer. 'No.'

'Then why? Why?' Miss Ruthie cried. 'I don't understand how you would know Ben married... and it never matter to you. What a selfish and terrible thing to do, Kat, your daddy turning in his grave. Blessed are those that walk in the shadow of the Almighty...'

There would be no benefit in trying to explain it to Miss Ruthie. Kat knew her mother saw things in black and white, good and bad, no middle ground, no excuses. But she had to try.

'I didn't know at first, Miss Ruthie, I swear to you. And I can't explain or tell you why I let it go so far.' The tears had not stopped, they were flowing heavier now. 'I love him, Miss Ruthie and he loves me too. We didn't want to hurt anyone.'

Miss Ruthie remained unforgiving. 'So you think because you love each other, it make it right to commit adultery?'

'No, it's not right,' Kat answered. 'But loving made it right for me.' She wiped her tears in frustration. 'Do you even know how hard it is? I wish I could just stop loving him at will, but how? Tell me how without ripping my own heart out, tell me and let me do it.'

'He has children too! Oh dear Lord, what a mess, what a mess. The shame, the shame, the shame!' Miss Ruthie stood to her feet, ranting. 'You need to stop all this now!' She clapped her hands firmly in quick succession. 'Put a stop to it, you hear me. If Ben was serious about you, he would be with you and Shadrach now, not with his wife and children. You were very, very foolish to think anything good could come of this.'

'I love him.' Kat turned her head away, heaving. She cried because no-one would understand what they had.

Miss Ruthie used an index finger to touch her child's chin, turning her to face her. 'I'm not against you but I'm disappointed. You must know it's wrong what you and Ben did. You have to let him go.'

Kat shook her head vigorously. 'I can't.'

'You must—he was never really yours.'

Forty-five

Ben

The familiar tropical heat welcomed Ben as he exited the plane at Montego Bay. The children had stayed with Auntie Joan because Claire had not returned home or answered any of his calls in two days, calling only to speak to the children and hanging up when he took the phone. It was obvious that her mother knew where she was, but took great pleasure in not telling.

It was late afternoon and the pre-booked taxi was waiting once he came through immigration. The drive to the Meadows seemed shorter than he remembered. A lot had changed in the months he had been away. Some of the dirt roads were replaced by tarmac; the town centre housed a Burger King and an Island Grill and halfway up the hill to Meadow View, the taxi driver told him, a drive-in cinema was being built.

He stayed at Meadows Inn, the same guest house he occupied on previous occasions and the following morning he strolled into town and signalled a passing taxi to stop. He climbed in without a glance at the driver.

'The Meadows,' he ordered, winding down the window.

'Mr Ben! It's you!'

Ben turned his head to the familiar voice and broke out in a smile. 'Dollar-Galore! What are you doing driving a taxi? Have you got a licence?'

The teenager beamed. 'Yes sah, my uncle buy me it,' he said proudly.

'Bought it for you? I thought you had to pass a test to get it.'

'With money you can buy anything in Jamaica, sah.'

Ben's frown was accompanied with a light-hearted chuckle. 'So I'm putting my life in the hands of a teenager who bought his driving licence, I'm not sure I should trust you.'

'I'm nineteen now, sah, and I been driving for nearly three years. Me is one safe driver, trust me.'

Ben relented. 'I don't want any foreigner prices... and I'm paying in Jamaican dollars.'

Galore's tone was heavy with disappointment. 'Alright, sah, but only because you and me is bredren and I never forget the trainers you buy us.' He drove on, steady.

Halfway up the hill the tarmac turned to dirt and rocks again and the drive became bumpy.

'No politicians don't live up here, so no need to fix the road.' Galore glanced at Ben in the back seat. 'You going to see Kat and Shaddy?'

Ben peered at him in the mirror. 'You know who I am to them?'

'Yes, man. Everyone does. Shaddy is my little friend. Bwoy, him look just like you. You couldn't deny him... you here for Kat, to take her back with you?'

'You think I should?'

'Yes, man, Kat deserves good. She have one of the sweetest hearts I know and a really great gyal to be around. My big Brother, Curtis, he use to hold a ting for her, you know, like her like that.' He looked in his front mirror, catching Ben's eyes, and laughed. 'But nothing came of that, my mother warn him off, tell him that Kat won't live long cause she have the sickness like her daddy, you know, her blood sick. But she still alive and even have baby, which I swear everyone thought she never could.' He had to break sudden, sending Ben forward as the car from the left cut in sharply.

'Hey, you see that idiot! Fool! Get him out a car mi mash up him...' he trailed as his eyes once again caught Ben's.

Ben listened thirstily, only now realising that there was so much he didn't know about Kat, they didn't know about each other.

'Yes, Miss Kat is a gem and I wish her all the best. She never have a bad word for anyone, except Nellie Potato and everyone have a bad word for that woman. I wonder though,' Galore seemed to have gone off in his own thoughts, 'whether she will be really happy, you know, really happy away from the Meadows. She love it so much. She love the sand, the sea, she love the rivers, she love the sun, she know 'bout the powers of the River Goddesses, she deep, you know. She deserves someone who can make her happy and love her like a woman likes to be loved. And I think you can. You can make her happy. My brother Curtis would keep other women alongside her, that's how he is and I feel that would kill her inside. You though can make her dreams come true. You wouldn't break her heart, mess with her, keep other women with her, she would be safe with you.'

Galore's banter seeped in like unwanted water into a boat. Ben was gripped by panic. He couldn't offer any of those. She was lost to him.

'Actually, I forgot something at the guest house, can you drop me back there now please.'

'Turn round? We nearly reach the house.'

'Turn around now!' The sharpness of Ben's voice made Galore break abruptly. He turned around to view his passenger for seriousness.

'Alright, alright. You paying and he who pays the piper calls the tune.'

The drive back to the guest house was accompanied by silence. Galore had a few attempts at conversation, but it was totally one-sided. At the end of the journey Ben paid and added a healthy tip.

'Thank you, sah,' Galore beamed. 'I don't know what I said to make you turn back, but sorry. My mother always tells me, "he who keepeth his mouth, keepth his life" but my mouth still run ahead of me.'

Ben could not speak; he got out of the car and walked into the guest house without a backward glance or a response to Galore's goodbyes.

He looked at his watch, it was almost seven. What was he doing? What could he tell Kat for sure? What was he here to offer? He walked out of the guest house again and Galore pulled up with a screech just as he exited the gates.

'I'll take you, free of charge, sah, anywhere you want to go.'

Ben watched as Miss Ruthie scattered corn for the

chickens in the front yard. She moved slowly and turned to look at the taxi that had pulled up. Ben got out and waved, opening the gate and she relaxed as recognition lit her face like a light bulb. As if remembering the recent events, she grew serious.

'Mr Ben, what you doing here? Kat know you coming? Only she gone down to the beach.'

'Hello, Miss Ruthie, it's nice seeing you again. No, I didn't tell her I was coming. How are you?'

'Oh, poor me dead woman child—but Sweet Jesus is merciful and I'm still here. Shaddy is inside, I leave him in the play pen because he get into all kind of mischief—he trying to stand now you know.'

Ben smiled. 'Yes, Kat told me. Can I go see him?'

'Go see him,' she ushered him with a stern hand movement.

He came back outside with the toddler in his arms. 'He's grown so big!' he exclaimed, grinning.

'And troublesome,' Miss Ruthie said with a proud smile.

Ben placed his son to stand, and with that Shadrach promptly fell on his nappy-padded bottom, making noises and attempts to follow the chickens.

'He like terrorising the animals so much, always shouting after them,' Miss Ruthie laughed.

Ben followed as Shadrach crawled slowly around the yard, stopping to pick up anything that caught his eyes, which Ben then had to take out of his hands before the child could stuff it into his mouth.

Finally he picked him up and joined Miss Ruthie, who was now sitting on the veranda, two glasses of lemonade and Shadrach's bottle on the table.

After closing the gate to the veranda, he sat down and sipped the lemonade thankfully.

'So,' Miss Ruthie said, reaching for her familiar brown bag of uncooked rice. 'What wind blew you this way?'

Ben sighed. 'The truth?' He didn't see any reasons to lie. 'I followed my heart.'

'Shouldn't your heart be with your wife? I know you married,' Miss Ruthie told him with her disapproving voice and look. 'I must tell you that I feel disappointment bad.'

'Miss Ruthie,' Ben said, 'it's all so complicated, but I love and respect Kat very much—'

'I not saying you don't, but you have a wife and children—I'm against fornication, it is a sin and it cannot go on.'

They were interrupted by the honk of a vehicle's horn as the jeep pulled up outside the gate. A figure carrying a huge package that partly blocked his view fumbled to open the gate without dropping the item. From the packaging, it was clear to see that it was a tricycle.

'It's Columbus,' Miss Ruthie whispered with a note of warning in her voice.

'*Bonjour*, good morning, Miss Ruthie.' He placed the box down before removing his large round spectacles. He rubbed them with the bottom of his tattered T-shirt. The sun had reddened his face and the thin white outline left by his glasses rendered him comical.

'Columbus, come join us.'

Ben stood to his feet; Shadrach in one arm and extended a hand of welcome.

'I'm—'

'I know who you are.' Columbus lips tightened

with control as he looked at Ben's outstretched hand as though it was offered for an examination and ignored it. A deafening silence swept the small veranda. Columbus eyed Ben venomously. Miss Ruthie crunched on her rice looking cautiously from Ben to Columbus and began to rock the chair gently, humming.

'Mr Ben come to see Shaddy—a surprise visit,' she told Columbus too brightly.

'Did he now?' Columbus said with obvious displeasure. Ben became aware of his French accent. 'Kat isn't one for surprises,' Columbus said looking at Miss Ruthie, but aiming the comment at Ben.

'I'm not here to—'

Columbus was quick to interrupt. 'What are you here for? Why have you come?'

The questions caused Ben's mind to reel. He did not want to ruin Kat's life, to leave her feeling rejected. He found himself thinking that maybe he had subliminally hitched a ride on the back of her dream. Her dream for a child was as acute as his for a son, if not more. There was something magical, something of a miracle in the child they had conceived and he now, like Kat, believed that their meeting was fate.

Miss Ruthie shifted stiffly in the rocking chair, sighing heavily. She crunched thoughtfully. Ben saw her eyes fill with mischief, drip by drip, like an unruly leak. 'I think Mr Ben have a right to come visit him son, Columbus. We can't deny a father the right to see him child.'

Columbus ran his hand nervously through his hair.

'Why?' Columbus spoke sternly. 'Kat does not want him here.'

Ben looked at him sharply. He was beginning to

366

feel annoyed, to resent this new age-looking creature before him.

'She loved surprises with me,' Ben announced evenly.

He saw the pulse throb in Columbus's jaws as he fought for some kind of control. Miss Ruthie saw it too.

'Lighten up, Columbus, you look as mad as a bull in a pen.'

'That is because I do not know what he is doing here.' He pointed with anger at Ben. 'Why come now? All the months Kat needed you and you were not here. I have always been here for her and Shaddy, you have no right coming here after what you did.'

Ben shook his head, as though trying to dislodge something. 'What I did?' He was clearly puzzled. 'What am I supposed to have done, in your opinion?'

Columbus fumed; his face and neck turning pink as he struggled with some volcanic force which could not be vocalised.

Ben's tone softened, 'I'm not here to justify my relationship with Kat. I'm not here to defend myself against any crime. There's so much I don't know about her, what she went through, her health, about her everyday life. I realise I know so little about her.' He looked at Miss Ruthie before returning his gaze to Columbus. 'But it didn't stop me from loving her because what I know is she... she's a great debater who loves red pea soup with coconut milk; she loves to walk the beach and feel the grains of sand between her toes. She loves to sit and watch the sunset—feel the breeze on her face and her favourite flower is baby's breath.' He watched Columbus' face turn pink with anger and knew he was twisting a knife in a wound, but he could not stop himself. He felt the need to let this man know just how deep he and Kat delved into each other.

'She's funny and laughs a lot and thinks about the stars and other universes. There's an answer for every question in her world, and when we went to the river, we had to give something to the river Goddess or she'd take it from us. She can smell rain coming and believes in Mother Cynthy and predictions. I fell in love with her and her kind of crazy.'

The silence settled like mist, even touching the squeaky rocking chair Miss Ruthie sat in. Ben watched the fight leave Columbus like a deflated rubber, his gaunt face transparent with anguish, his thin lips trembling with emotions. It was hard to conceal the sympathy that suddenly stirred in the pit of his stomach as he watched Columbus. He knew now how much Kat meant to him and if he could have done it any other way, he would, for it would have been humane to avoid inflicting any more pain.

'Why have you come? What do you want?' Columbus pushed the words out between gritted teeth. 'What do you want?' Columbus demanded again.

'Kat,' Ben said simply.

Forty-six .
Kat

The sun was hot and still. Quietness saturated the terrain until the sound of nature tunnelled in with the ruffles of dry falling leaves as the breeze whipped by. The tweeting birds, the buzzing bees and barking dogs drifted towards her. She lay on her back, eyes closed savouring the warmth of the sun on her face and revelling in the peace that bathed her. If only she could make this feeling last. But she knew once she left the serenity of this surrounding, the confusion would return.

Something touched her forehead, causing her to open her eyes just in time to see the erratic flight of a black, yellow and red butterfly. She squinted as an object in the distance, over the other side of the river bank caught her attention. She couldn't remember seeing it before and knew it must be a new addition. It was a statue of a family of dolphins, mother, father and baby in the middle. She thought of Claire and wondered if she had gone home. She hoped so. The thought that she might still be in the Meadows unnerved her. All that anger, the pain, it haunted her to think of Claire's eyes, to live through her words again. *I am Mrs Thornton Benjamin, who are you?* She had almost ran out of the restaurant leaving that question unanswered. The truth of it lingered worse than any bee sting she had ever had. The dancing butterfly kept returning to her, scooping her attention as it now danced around the stone dolphins.

'Kat.' She bolted upright at the familiar sound of the voice. Turning around she saw it was Mother Cynthy.

'I went down to the beach but never find you—I know the next place to look is the river.'

'What is it, Mother Cynthy?' Kat was alarmed to see the old lady so far from her usual route.

'Kat,' she breathed, 'when rain's going to fall, you close your windows.'

'What?'

'When trouble coming step aside.'

Kat's eyes clouded with the thought of Claire-Louise. Mother Cynthy was immediate with her observation.

'Trouble come already, I see.' She nodded knowingly. 'I hope you dealt with it wisely.'

The peace that had engaged Kat evaporated like smoke on a breezy day. The roller coaster had started and gathered speed. She didn't want to think about Claire or the elderly English gentleman she met who had unknowingly thrown another light, giving a different shade to things. She considered it divine, their meeting, and he was so sure his daughter would be leaving Nellie Potato's married grandson, so sure of her, but if she loved him like she loved Ben, how could she leave him? Kat wanted to know.

'Love demands great sacrifices. It does,' Mother Cynthy said purposely.

Kat stood up and brushed the debris of nature from

her clothing. Why now? Why did people have to come and stir doubt?

'You know something, Mother Cynthy. You know something which you're not telling me. What else did you see?'

'You take a journey. And there's struggle ahead but it will be for the best, many doors will open for you. I see greatness if you follow your heart, that first thought.'

Mother Cynthy left as suddenly as she came.

Kat walked to the front entrance of the gardens where taxis waited for their daily fares. She was in turmoil as the taxi drove towards her home, and it was nearing sunset by the time she finally arrived. Miss Ruthie would not be too pleased at all the hours she had been gone and she braced herself for the dressing down she knew would come.

It was unusual not to see Miss Ruthie on the veranda in her rocking chair with the brown paper bag of rice on the small table beside her, and not a flicker of light. As she climbed the stairs her heart quickened as the thought rapidly drifted through her mind that perhaps Miss Ruthie was feeling unwell or something had happened to Old Man or Shaddy. That would be the only thing to prevent her from sitting on her beloved veranda watching the sunset. She opened the door and walked into the dining area, only to see Columbus sitting at the table in the darkness.

'Col, what's wrong? Where's Miss Ruthie and Old Man? Where's Shaddy?' Her voice held the panic she felt. Turning on the light and observing his face, fear gripped her. 'What's wrong? Where's everyone?'

'They've gone for a drive.'

She became puzzled. 'A drive? Where to?' She pulled out a chair and sat facing him.

He reached for her hand across the table and squeezed them gently. She saw anguish in his eyes.

'Col, what is going on? Why you looking like that?'

His face gave way to a smile that did not reach his eyes. '*Je veux que tu saches que tu es la seule femme que j'ai jamais aimé...* I want you to know that you are the only woman I have ever loved... apart from my mother. From the moment I met you I loved you—you do know that, don't you?'

'Col, you're starting to sound like a mad man. What's wrong?'

He brought her hands to his lips and kissed them. He went on kissing them until she gently pulled away.

'Col, talk to me. I'm feeling that something isn't quite right. Are you sick?'

He laughed. 'That would be easy.'

'Then what's not easy?'

He stood to his feet and tucked his hands into his pocket. '*L'amour...* love.'

'Col! What's got into you?'

Kat had known her friend for far too long not to know when something was seriously wrong. She stood up and walked the few steps to stand before him. She circled his waist with her arms and hugged him affectionately.

'Talk to me, friend. We've always been honest with each other, let's not start anything different now.'

'Yes, let's not.'

She moved away, but stayed close enough for her hands to rest on his waist. 'What gripe you, Col?'

372

'Ben... your lover, the only man you love... the father of your son.'

Her hands dropped and she took a step back, her eyes now digging into his.

'What's your gripe, Col?' she repeated, now sterner.

'I think I've been fooling myself—'

'Fooling yourself?'

'Yes, because I've been thinking, why couldn't I have been the man from across the ocean... been thinking that one day, maybe you might–might love me.'

Kat looked hopelessly at him. She had never known him to be like this. In all the years they had been friends, never stepping over the invisible boundaries they both knew were in place.

He sat down again, removing his glasses and burying his head in the crook of his arm. She went to him and stroked his hair knowing she could not comfort him.

'I'm so sorry, friend. I was wrong, so wrong about so many things, or maybe I just closed my mind to them... I feel so conflicted, I'm crying all the time—'

'He is here for you. He has come back for you and Shaddy... he is here now... come to steal you... *il est ici, là pour toi*... he's come for you. Ben.'

Forty-seven
Kat

The house suddenly felt far too hot, too stuffy to be inside. Kat walked out onto the veranda and sat in her chair. Columbus followed a few minutes later. Ben was back in Jamaica and according to Columbus had come back for her and Shadrach. Had he made his choice? Mother Cynthy had said she would take a journey, great things lay ahead. Turmoil embroiled her, throwing her into a pool of confusion with no branch to hold on to. Ben. The very thought of him churned her abdomen, fluttered her heart, made her think of passion between white cotton sheets, of love on the beach, of how much she had held down, held back the thought of him. Now it was twirling her into a tsunami and all she could do to keep sane was to stay quiet. Not utter a word.

Columbus stood close to her, his presence suddenly claustrophobic; his words running havoc in her head and with Claire and the elder still fresh on her mind.

'What now?' Columbus's voice was quiet and scared. She felt terrible because she could offer him no comfort.

'I–I don't know. I'll have to wait and see what Ben... says.'

'And then?'

'I don't know what he'll say.'

He sat down in Miss Ruthie's chair so that he could see her face. 'If he says he will leave his wife and children for you? Would that be okay?'

'Col, you've been there for me through thick and thin. Many times I opened my eyes in a hospital bed and it's your face I saw, your voice I heard. Then you've been so good for Shaddy, I can't forget those things. I owe you. But don't judge me. And don't ask me any questions that I can't give you answers to—let me speak with Ben first.'

'Owe me? Owe me? Speak to Ben first?' A dry burst of laughter left his lips. 'I wish you could just fall in love with me... but that will not happen, will it?' He looked offended.

She wasn't going to lie. 'No, Col. That would eventually destroy you... and me.'

He interrupted her, 'What about Ben? He told me that he was here for you... for Shaddy. He's leaving his wife and children, *il est venu pour toi*... He wants you, Kat.'

The thought made joy riot within her momentarily, long enough for Columbus to see.

'It makes me sad that I can't be happy for you on this one.'

'I'm sorry.'

'Me too, me too.' He bent to kiss her forehead then left, driving off at speed in his jeep, leaving a trail of dust behind him.

Miss Ruthie and Old Man arrived an hour later, but it

was the figure walking in behind them that made Kat's heart skip. Ben, with Shadrach asleep in his arms. Kat held onto every ounce of control not to throw herself at him. He looked at her wearily.

'Hey, you.'

This was too much. She felt the tears well up and there was nothing she could do to stop them from rolling down her face. Miss Ruthie took Shadrach before she and Old Man made themselves scarce. 'I'll put this sleepy baby to bed,' she said.

Kat looked into Ben's eyes and drew a sharp breath. Such transparency. Love was staring back at her.

'I didn't know you were coming,' she sniffed.

'I know. It was the only way I could do this.'

'What exactly are you doing?'

He pulled up the stool and sat down, patting her tears with a handkerchief before giving it to her. She wiped the tears away hurriedly, her raised eyebrows arched with unvoiced questions.

'Claire is mad... it was she who took Miss Ruthie's phone call, it made her aware of Shaddy. You see, we always wanted a son and earlier this year things went bad and she had an ectopic.'

'I am sorry to hear that. Claire actually called me and I met with her at Hotel Panama.'

Ben's eyes opened alarmingly. 'She was in Jamaica? She came?'

Kat nodded, noticing how crushed he looked and she felt the need to cry, to hold him and apologise for messing up his life.

'Yes.'

'She gave you a hard time? What did she say?'

'Told me how much she loves her husband, that she's the only Mrs Benjamin, who the fuck am I? And she's right, we both know that.'

'She can have a mouth on her, but she has a soft centre. You changed my life, Kat and nothing is the same. Finding out about Shaddy, I guess it changed me from the husband she knew. I've come and I don't know what I'm going to say to you. All I know for sure is that I ache for you.'

'What do you do about it?'

His eyes misted with bleakness and she had to fight the urge not to rush into his arms.

'I'm in love with you, Kat.'

She stood up and looked towards the gate that beckoned her to run, to leave this mess she had created behind. She became agitated.

'In the beginning we said we wouldn't let what we have hurt anyone—now we've destroyed Claire-Louise. I love you, Ben, very much and if love was all that's needed, I could be yours this instant.' She clicked her fingers close to his eyes. 'But it isn't. There's more to relationships than love.'

'Like what?' he demanded.

'Like not being wrong and strong. We went into love with both eyes open but we were only looking at each other, not at your wife... or your children. We got lost in the moment and carried away by our wants and it was good, oh God, it was good. But now we got to be real.'

'Miss Ruthie and Old Man spoke to me about that too,' Ben admitted. 'I told them this feeling I have inside for you, it has a will all of its own, I'm weak to it.'

'Me too,' she confessed, 'but I have to find the strength.'

'To leave me?'

'Yes.'

'Really?'

'Yes.'

'Are you serious? I can't challenge this?'

'You'd never win.'

'What about Shaddy? I want him to know me; I want to be in his life, you have no idea how much. He's my son... my son!'

'You can be in his life. There's no reason why he can't visit you during the holidays. I want him to know you too.'

'And what will you do? I'm selfish, I can't bear the thought of you with anyone else.'

She sighed. 'Don't, Ben. Be nice and let me go.'

'I can't.'

'You must.'

'Why?'

'Because this is our karma. Your wife needs you and you know it's the right thing to do. Can you imagine how she bleeds inside her heart? Knowing you betrayed her with another woman who gave you a son... we didn't mean to, but we messed up badly. Now we can be truthful to ourselves, we know this ending was inevitable. Even like you say, you love us both; I should have known that with love so equal, you would have to go with the one you loved the longest. There must be some equation in the universe that makes that right.'

She watched him stand up and walk to stand close to her, taking her hands in his, smiling through his tears.

'Blame it on the universe. I somehow knew you'd be the one to end it, you hide so much from me and this is my karma—you don't need me.'

Her breath caught in her throat, along with the protest she wanted to holler out.

'Claire doesn't want me,' he told her earnestly. 'I've hurt her so badly, she may never forgive me.'

Kat turned to face him, her eyes fighting with tears but her mouth fixed with determination.

'Deep down you can't possibly believe that, Ben. You must know that pain causes us to speak irrationally. We use words as weapons to wound and protect ourselves from any force that threatens to harm our world. Claire-Louise was hoping you loved her enough to fight for her; she doesn't want you gone, she only wanted to see if you would fight to stay. Look what she gave me for Shaddy. She was so angry with me, hated me, but she gave me this for our son.'

Kat saw Ben's eyes mist over before he closed them and she knew, he knew what the Man U tracksuit she held up meant. When his eyes opened the tears were up to the brim, and ran down his cheeks with a blink.

The truth swims like oil on top of water. No matter how much you splash to disturb that oil to prevent it from being seen, its various shapes find themselves together as sure as a magnet finds steel.

'She is amazing. Claire is amazing and I love her, I love her so much, but I love you no less. I'm not choosing her over you, you must believe that. I would never reject you.' It was a plea, a prayer of sorts as he lifted her hand to his lips, kissing the soft tips of her fingers.

Her blink was not quick enough to barricade the tears and when she opened her eyes, the tears met her trembling lips.

'I know, Ben. Left to you like Claire-Louise said, you'd have us both because you don't want to let any of us down. Thanks for the love, it was beautiful, it was real and it gave me our son.'

'It was fate, right?'

She smiled. 'You can't tell me different.'

His movement was impulsive as he bent his head to kiss her. She didn't move and he kissed her, lingeringly.

'You're my love, Kat,' he breathed, sipping her neck and the familiar ripples of desire stirred in that most intimate part of her body until she gently untangled herself.

She cupped his damp face with both hands and kissed him again, her lips trembling with the weight of the hurt.

'I wanted you to choose me. I wanted you for me and Shaddy, but we wouldn't have been happy that way. We would have no peace knowing what we did to your wife and children. I can't believe how selfish I was. Love demands sacrifices and I'm strong enough to make them, Ben. How dare we think just because we love each other we can do what we want! We can't. We can't. There's more to consider than just "us", and we still have time to make it better... eventually.'

Forty-seven
Kat

The following morning Kat arrived at the hotel with Shadrach. Her heart twisted when she saw Ben's eyes that had been deprived of sleep by a hurricane passing through, leaving behind the debris of misery. It was the hardest thing not to fall into him and tell him that she wanted to be his.

'Hey, sweet girl.' His smile was a shadow that barely crossed his lips. He held out his arms to Shadrach, who went willingly with that wide smile of recognition babies have on seeing familiar faces.

'If you can drop him home before sunset—he likes to have his bath before then, and it settles him more for the night.'

'No problem... you coming in? Want to join us for the day out?' Ben asked, eyes pleading.

'Not this time.'

He nodded, visibly understanding. 'See you later then.'

'Okay,' she turned quickly to walk away.

'It's too hard to let you go; can you let me go so easily?'

She turned around to look at him. 'It's the hardest thing I've ever done, and it hurts badly that we can't have each other, but there's no alternative. We now know that. This is our karma.'

And to think it all started with Mother Cynthy's prediction... of her swimming with fishes.

Kat knew when he arrived at sunset she could not be there—she did not trust herself to see him again without yielding to him. Not for now. Life would be dismal for a while, to wake each day knowing that it was all over would take time, a great deal of time before her heart would beat smooth again. The task that lay ahead of her was colossal. Mother Cynthy had been right. Love truly demands great sacrifices.

Outside, Rosie and Ras Solomon sat in their old Honda truck waiting for her.

'What you gonna do now?' Rosie asked.

'I phoned Paula the other day; I'm going to take her up on her offer to visit Namibia. I'm going on a journey. She even thinks I can get a job teaching art in schools once I sort out my visa, and she's a stay at home mum so she'll look after Shaddy.'

'You going Africa? Not on Miss Rootie's watch, you mad? You betta tell her it in a letter which she can read when you on the plane, and the plane must have taken off.'

Kat smiled. 'I've made up my mind. Just for a year or so, or maybe longer. I have to find a place to put all of this. My life is forever changed, and so am I.' Her voice broke.

'You okay?' Rosie's face was full of sympathy.

Kat pulled deeply for a smile and patted Rosie's hand. 'No, no, but borrowing Miss Ruthie's phrase; I will be... with time that great healer.'

Acknowledgements

I'd first like to thank my four sons, who always encouraged me and allowed me the precious time to write.

To Femi Odufunade, thank you for the glimpse into your world as a sickle cell sufferer. Darling Marcelle Roujade, so grateful for your time and energy spent translating my French narrative around my kitchen table, LOL. To the JustWrite Creative Writing Group for all the feedbacks, creativity and the fun. To the remarkable women and men who touched my life, coloured it with your stories... I love you all, so many to name, but you know who you are.

As ever, love and thanks to Jacaranda Books, I am incredibly blessed to have the support of such an awesome team—thank you Valerie Brandes and Laure Deprez, for assisting my dream from pen to shelf. Thank you, authors, Sareeta Domingo and Irenosen Okojie for enhancing my knowledge and my craft.

For Albert Feeney (Mr Feeney), my English teacher at Highfield School Letchworth, who wrote in my final year report; 'A brilliant author who hides her light under a bushel.' I never knew what you meant then, Mr Feeney, but now I do and I have never forgotten you or those words.

Finally... to my world of girls, sister-friends... you fill my soul with your laughter and your stories.

About the Author

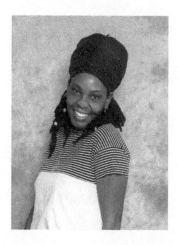

Rasheda Ashanti Malcolm is a writer, playwright and radio presenter. She has been rewarded by many prizes, including the Black Business Woman of the Year, the National Black Women Achievement Award and more recently, the Pandora Award for Publishing. Rasheda's first novel was a runner-up in the Saga Literary Prize. She initiated the Candace Black Women Achievement Award, and is the co-founder of WILDE International Network. She currently teaches Creative Writing in London and is a Gender Abuse Consultant.

About the Author